An Illustrated Guide to
TAPING TECHNIQUES

Commissioning Editor: Claire Wilson
Development Editor: Ewan Halley and Fiona Conn
Project Manager: Elouise Ball
Designer: Kirsteen Wright
Illustration Manager: Bruce Hogarth

An Illustrated Guide to
TAPING TECHNIQUES
Principles and Practice

SECOND EDITION

Tom Hewetson
MSc BSc (Hons) Ost Med
Principal Osteopath of the Osteopathic Clinic Ltd
London, UK

Karin A. Austin
BPT BSc (Ph Th)
Consultant
Physiotherapie Internationale KA Inc
Montreal, Canada

Kathryn A. Gwynn-Brett
BSc (PT), Dip MI
Sole Charge Physiotherapist
Mississauga Orthopaedic and Sports Injury Clinic,
Canada

Sarah C. Marshall
BSc (PT), MSc (Rehab Sci)
Physiotherapist
Ste-Anne's Hospital
Ste-Anne de Belleuue, Canada

Forewords by:
Lynn Booth
MCSP MSc
Chartered Physiotherapist, UK

Jonathan Betser
DO
Osteopathic Sports Care Consultant
Clinical Director, Woodside Clinic
Chairman, Osteopathic Sports Care Association, UK

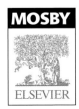
MOSBY
ELSEVIER

Edinburgh   London   New York   Oxford   Philadelphia   St Louis   Sydney   Toronto   2010

MOSBY
ELSEVIER

ISBN 978 0723 43482 5

British Library Cataloguing in Publication Data
A catalogue record for this book is available from the British Library

Library of Congress Cataloging in Publication Data
A catalog record for this book is available from the Library of Congress

ELSEVIER your source for books, journals and multimedia in the health sciences
www.elsevierhealth.com

Working together to grow
libraries in developing countries

www.elsevier.com | www.bookaid.org | www.sabre.org

ELSEVIER   BOOK AID International   Sabre Foundation

The publisher's policy is to use **paper manufactured from sustainable forests**

Printed in China

Contents

The DVD accompanying this text includes video clips of some commonly-used techniques and helpful tips. To look at the video, click on the relevant icon in the contents list on the DVD. The disc is designed to be viewed in conjunction with the text and not as a stand-alone product.

Preface

An Illustrated Guide to Taping Techniques: Principles and Practice is appropriate for use as:

- A textbook for medical and manual therapy courses, including physiotherapy, osteopathy, chiropractics, and sports therapy
- A guide for sports coaches
- A guide for emergency room staff
- A source of specific referenced material for any practitioner encountering patients who are employing the use of tape and for those practitioners who are applying tape.

Designed to accommodate the requirements of clinicians and their patients, this guide offers highly informative, clearly illustrated taping methods developed by persons actively involved in the care of patients, especially those in the athletic community where tape and supports are used on a regular basis. The authors' collective experience involves multiple aspects of patient care including education and clinical application, as well as active involvement as support personnel at national level and international level sporting events.

An authoritative comprehensive guide, *An Illustrated Guide to Taping Techniques: Principles and Practice* will prove indispensable to students from a wide range of clinical backgrounds including medicine, physiotherapy, osteopathy, chiropractic, sports therapy, as well as to sports coaches, trainers, physical educators, managers, and the athlete and their family. Students will learn the scientific principles that direct the application of tape. It is recommended as a teaching manual, as well as a practical guide in hospital emergency rooms, doctors' surgeries, sports injury clinics, physiotherapy centres, osteopathic and chiropractic clinics and on site at athletic events.

Essential to effective treatment and rehabilitation of injuries which need taping is an understanding of the type, mechanism and degree of injury, the tissues involved, the repair process as it applies to those tissues, the appropriate taping materials for the structure being dealt with, and the proper application

of those materials. Taping should be used in conjunction with treatment and a comprehensive rehabilitation program that is aimed at reducing inflammation and pain, restoring range of motion, flexibility, strength, and proprioception. Referring to this guide, the practitioner will be able to address complex situations by using the appropriate, effective techniques for providing adequate compression, stability and support to the injured structure. Whether the desired effect is immediate return to activity or gradual rehabilitation, once the injury has been properly assessed and diagnosed, correct application of the specific taping technique to the injured area will ensure protection and allow functional mobility.

This guide has been divided into two sections. Sections cover taping supplies with a general description of their characteristics and uses; principles of taping including taping guidelines with a unique review system using the acronyms **S.U.P.P.O.R.T.** and **P.R.E.C.A.U.T.I.O.N.**; charts for sprains, strains and contusions using the mnemonic T.E.S.T.S., plus an overview of various types of tape strips.

The second section covers taping techniques for specific injuries. Clear step-by-step photographs and detailed instructions guide the taper. A list of supplies and positioning relative to each taping application is included, and a simple injury assessment and treatment chart follows each technique.

The guide is supplemented by a DVD containing some commonly used techniques and helpful tips.

Once the information in this package has been assimilated and techniques practiced and mastered, the practitioner will have an excellent base on which to build their taping repertoire. Those involved in taping regularly will, through experience, develop the ability to adapt the principles and techniques in this guide to a myriad of situations.

Tom Hewetson
2010

Acknowledgements

The author would like to thank the following people for their assistance in completing this project:

Karin Austin, Kathryn Gwynn-Brett and Sarah Marshall for writing the first edition of this book and allowing me to update and add to their original work.

Jon McSwiney and Paul Graham who proof read and helped revise the final book.

Sarena Wolfaard, Claire Wilson and Claire Bonnett from Elsevier for commissioning this edition and asking me to contribute to it.

Grant Snowdon, a good friend who modelled for the photographs and the DVD.

Marc Broom, Photographer: from Timeless Photos Ltd.

Mark Slocombe, Creation Video.

The many experienced therapists who, over the years, have shared their techniques and knowledge, allowing us to learn and to develop and improve skills that can now be shared with others.

Professor Eyal Lederman, mentor and all round good guy, for his inspiration.

Finally, to my wife **Jayne** and daughters **Emma** and **Chloé** whose patience, love and encouragement have sustained me through the updating of this book and production of the accompanying DVD.

Heartfelt thanks to all

Foreword

The use of taping procedures within the sporting environment has increased over recent years; in part due to improved communication and exchange of ideas between practitioners, at home and abroad, who advocate different treatment practices and techniques. The improvement in the taping materials available has also allowed greater variety in techniques and hence provides a greater incentive to use taping procedures. The large variety of tape available enables the practitioner to adapt conventional techniques to ones that are more suitable for a particular injury and/or athlete. Taping procedures are used prophylactically, as a treatment modality and in order to give reassurance on returning to sport. In its different guises, it can be used with benefit through the full extent of injury management: providing compression or reducing unwanted movement/stress in the acute stage of an injury; providing proprioceptive feedback as treatment progresses; supporting injured structure(s) in a functional position during rehabilitation (thus enhancing confidence).

This book provides both the novice and the more experienced practitioner with an easy-to-read, clear and concise approach to taping many of the joints and soft tissues which may be injured during sport and exercise. In the past, a frequent criticism of taping procedures has been that it is helping to "prop up" injured tissues which should not be returning to sport or even to modified activity. The authors' use of continuous reminders within the book leaves the reader in no doubt that taping is no substitute for treatment/rehabilitation and should not be used without first fully assessing the injury and reaching a (working) diagnosis. In all injuries, an initial assessment, accurate diagnosis and on-going assessment of an injury are vital in gaining the best possible result.

Within the sporting environment, those involved in taping must be aware of the differing rules of competition for different sports. These rules vary from sport to sport, may change from year to year and may prohibit the use of tape to protect certain joints or may only permit a certain type and/or colour of tape to be used within competition.

Taping should be functional and should always achieve its objective without using excessive amounts of tape or causing too much disruption to surrounding tissues or to the athlete as a whole. The more discrete the tape, whilst doing its job, the more an athlete and/or patient will appreciate the intervention and the person who has applied it.

Taping is often deemed to be the preserve of the sporting population and those practitioners who work within sport. This book illustrates, by word and diagram, how appropriate taping is for many soft tissue injuries at various stages of the healing/recovery process, whether the injury has been caused during a sporting activity, an occupational activity or even just by an unfortunate accident. Taping can also be used regardless of the age of the injured person – providing, of course, their skin condition is suitable for taping to be used. The latter point is, of course, very relevant in a sporting environment when treating athletes with a disability.

The easy-to-understand diagrams and text enable the reader to replicate the taping procedures and, as experience is gained, to develop his/her own procedures using the basis of the techniques provided here. An injury can present in a variety of ways during the different stages of healing, treatment and rehabilitation. This text allows the practitioner to use imagination and discrimination regarding the movements which may have to be restricted and/or supported and the means to enable this to happen.

This book not only provides advice on taping application. It also provides a handy *aide-memoire* regarding surface anatomy and an outline of basic treatment protocols for common soft-tissue injuries.

As with all treatment modalities, "practice makes perfect" and this is certainly true of taping. A proficient practitioner can make a taping job look easy, it can be accomplished quickly with the minimal amount of fuss and the result is an effective, efficient taping job with no wrinkles, creases or exposed surfaces. When starting out using taping procedures, what is actually achieved is far from this ideal. The authors' recurring message regarding the need to practice is very important. There is nothing worse than spending a considerable time in applying tape only to have to remove it because it is ineffective or liable to cause more problems, for example if it compromises the skin condition or circulation. However, it is important that practitioners do not try to save face by deciding not to remove and reapply a poor taping job. This may save the practitioners' embarrassment but the athlete/patient will certainly not thank them in the end! If it is going wrong, stop and start again. As the authors emphasise, to avoid this embarrassment and delay practitioners must practice on a regular basis until each technique is smooth and they convey an air of confidence at all times. It goes without saying that anyone with an injury will always have more confidence in those who appear competent at their job.

All readers will find this book useful: whether they are novices who wish to learn the art of taping or more established practitioners who wish to refresh their memory or confirm an opinion.

Lynn Booth
2010

Foreword

As the excellent references and bibliography in this book demonstrate, there are numerous studies that have confirmed (and re-confirmed) the considerable benefit of effective taping and, as we all know, whether your working environment is clinic-based or pitchside/trackside, the judicious implementation of some functionally appropriate tape can, on occasions, change your treatment from 'appreciated pain relief' to a legitimate way to enable and enhance performance.

Protecting one's body is an obvious necessity in the heat of battle (whether sporting or military) - and taping and strapping have been the cornerstone of good sportscare management for as long as humans have been competitive and sports loving. Pictures from the ancient civilisations of Rome and Greece show us that (and if Achilles had managed to have better protection around his ankle, his place in history might be a very different one). One can imagine some long distant relative of Tom Hewetson managing to avoid the rigours of the gladiatorial arena with the same skills that Tom demonstrates in his lecture work and in this excellent update of an important book.

The Hewetson I know has, after all, been doing the same job with modern gladiators, such as rugby legend Lawrence Dallaglio, for the last 15 years. Like any committed professional should, Tom truly believes in doing the best job he can for each and every patient he sees. He's also passionate about the value offered by a genuinely inter-professional sports medicine team.

Although physiotherapists and athletic trainers have generally held dominion in the area of taping and strapping, with the application of the osteopathic principle of 'structure governs function', those osteopaths who work extensively with sportsmen and women have also found that they can very effectively integrate taping into their own (osteopathic approach) to treatment.

I'm delighted therefore that someone like Tom was approached to update *An Illustrated Guide to Taping Techniques*. The thorough way which the reader is taken through the principles, objectives and basic pathology which relate to taping, before being introduced to the anatomically specific taping techniques, offers an ideal introduction to those new to taping (and is ideal revision for those already experienced in the 'Art'!).The techniques that feature in the book will provide you with a great selection for you to 'dip into' on your taping journey. You must also use the DVD – taping is, after all, more than just theory! There can be no better way to learn good taping practice than to watch an expert in action, and Tom, although I hesitate to let him know that I think so, certainly is an expert.

So I urge you, don't just use this book for reference; read it from cover to cover! Embrace the considerable value that good taping and strapping can add to your treatment armoury (assuming you aren't already doing so), and you'll soon find yourself refining and developing these techniques, and your strapping and taping will rapidly evolve into an approach which incorporates your own unique 'take' on this wonderfully effective and useful skill.

My own opportunity to attain legendary status in the firmament of taping supremos was when I realised the value of medially fixing the patella when it was mal-tracking. Unfortunately (although this was before Jenny McConnell had published her ground-breaking article in *Australian Journal of Physiotherapy*), where I fell short was in the complexity of my (very!) long lever strapping and my technique's inability to allow the knee to flex more than 40 degrees (which made for an interesting tuck move in Trampolining!). Surprisingly, Jenny's evidence-based approach of applying just a couple of pieces of tape whilst allowing both re-alignment and re-education of a fully functional knee somehow proved more successful! That's why the rest of us need experts like Tom and Jenny – so we can learn from them and look good in front of our patients!

Well done, Tom – good job!

Jonathan Betser
2010

Introduction

The aims of the book and DVD are simple: they are designed as teaching aids for those looking to incorporate taping techniques in their work with patients or athletes, as well as a source of reference material for those who already employ taping techniques. At present there are few books on taping and even fewer that could be recommended as a reference book for teaching establishments. This book takes a comprehensive look at taping, the role of tape as a remedial and prophylactic tool, and other effects that applying tape can have.

The book lays out easy-to-read and understand tables of approaches to taping specific injured areas of the body. It uses unique acronyms and mnemonics in looking at specific injuries and gives general advice on how to approach treatment of those injuries, making the book user friendly.

The DVD is a visual guide to a range of techniques and is designed to be complementary to the book.

Athletic taping is the most common type of taping technique used. It uses a rigid or semi rigid form of tape that is designed to be used for the duration of a sport and then removed. This type of taping is predominantly, but not exclusively, used in the athletic community because it is an excellent tool that can be used as part of a comprehensive treatment and rehabilitation regime, that may enable the athlete to return to activity with the assistance and support that tape can offer. It is essential that one should always thoroughly assess and evaluate an injury, or make sure that an injury has been thoroughly assessed and diagnosed prior to taping. However, there are certain techniques that can be used as a form of protection, such as a sling, while awaiting a proper examination and diagnosis.

We must always remember that the application of tape will have physiological, biomechanical, neuro-physiological and psychological ramifications, and that it should never be applied without taking these considerations into account. It is not as simple as applying a piece of sticky tape or a support bandage to someone. There has to be a clinical reason for applying the tape. According to Frett and Reilly[1], improper taping or taping for no reason may predispose an athlete to injury or add to the severity of an existing injury.

Tape, strapping, braces and supports have been used for many years and for many reasons. Below are some of the reasons for using various forms of taping:

- to hold wound dressings in place, as in simple bandaging
- to compress injury sites during the acute or inflammatory phase of an injury to help decrease inflammatory exudates and their irritating effects
- to offer support to an injury site, either as an initial form of protection until a full examination can be carried out (for example, whilst the patient is being transported to the emergency room) or to support the injured structures between initial treatments minimizing the extent of the injury
- to support these injured structures during rehabilitation, especially when the athlete can return to controlled activities and thus maintain his fitness level and skills while avoiding exacerbation of the injury
- to continue to support prophilactically, after an area has been treated and rehabilitated and the patient has returned to normal activities. This approach offers the region continued support and may decrease the chance of re-injury[2-7].

The contemporary usefulness of these materials:

- Affects neuromotor control, by altering joint mechanics [8-13]
- Affects proprioceptive feedback and assist in restoration of balance [14-21]
- Assists in pain management by affecting joint range of motion, decrease the effects of inflammatory exudates and to off-load pain producing tissues [22-26]

Tapes are used in hospital emergency rooms, doctor's surgeries, physiotherapy, osteopathic, chiropractic, sports injury therapy practices and practically every sports club in the world.

The key to any successful taping technique will involve to a greater or lesser degree, several factors, such as:

- **An understanding of the mechanism of injury / pathogenesis**

  All the answers are in the case history. As long as they were compos mentis at the time of injury, the athlete will generally tell you how the injury occurred. Remember to ask for specifics. Any patient will tell you where the pain is, the lateral ankle for example, and tell you how it happened (e.g. playing football), but you will need specifics in order to work out exactly what has happened and is likely to be happening to what tissues. Ask them exactly how it happened. This will allow you to work out the possible structures damaged. At this point, you are probably thinking that they have twisted the ankle (an inversion injury) and damaged the anterior talo-fibular ligament. This is a reasonable assumption to make, as the ankle is a commonly injured site and this is the most common type of ankle injury[27, 28, 29] and probably the most common mechanism of injuring the lateral ankle. However, what if they tell you that it was not twisted, and that someone jumped on it? This should bring to mind different possibilities for structures injured. The answers to your questions should lead you to perform relevant clinical tests which should then guide you to a diagnosis or suggest when to refer for specific tests such as Ultrasound scan, X-ray, CT or MRI scan, or referral on to a third party.

- **An understanding of the pathophysiology and extent of the injury**

  Understanding the degree of damage to the tissues will determine the type of treatment and amount of assistance the patient will need from tape. There is ambiguity on consensus on classifying the extent of a soft tissue injury. Generally, a grade one injury is a mild injury with no tearing or laxity of the tissue, a grade two injury is a mild to moderate injury with some tissue tearing and laxity, and a grade three is a moderate to severe with substantial tearing and laxity to a complete rupture of the tissues[30-32]. Why do we want to grade the injury? Unless we know the approximate damage caused we cannot reasonably work out a treatment and rehabilitation regime for the patient, or to what extent we should tape. You could end up not doing enough taping or doing too much. This may be a problem as, with the former, the injury may be prolonged at best, exacerbated at worst, and with the latter may go on to create a new problem as too much immobility may lead to other tissue changes [28-31]. Also, you can give an approximate time of recovery to the patient [32, 33].

- **An understanding of the general repair process as it applies to the tissues injured**

  As the injury responds to treatment and recovers so the athlete will need less support from tape. Having an understanding of the repair process and what happens in each phase of repair will assist you to make the decision when to use more or less support, as the case may be. For example, what technique you should use in what phase. Initially, during the inflammatory or acute phase (phase 1) you may want to use a compression technique to assist in limiting swelling. In the proliferative, matrix or regeneration phase (phase 2) you may want to use a technique that will offer plenty of support limiting full range of motion. During the remodelling phase (phase 3) you may want to choose techniques that will be less restrictive but still supportive and assists in the limitation of pain.

  Having knowledge of the approximate rates at which tissues repair [32, 33] should help you inform the athlete of, approximately, how long they can expect to be taped. This, of course, will depend on the extent of damage. Remember, these times are arbitrary time scales and as different tissues repair at different rates so will different patients. Depending on the extent of the injury, repair can range from several days to several months[36, 37]. The cells of tissue repair have been found in and around an injury site up to 12 months after it was deemed the injury had recovered[38]. It is therefore better to use the athlete's ability and pain as a guide to recovery.

- **An understanding of the functional anatomy of the area to be taped**

  In reality, if you know the functional anatomy (the structures and normal range of motion) of the injured region and what ranges of motion are to be limited, you could have a reasonable attempt without tuition at applying tape to limit those ranges of motion. However, with tuition and guidance on what tape and accessories to use in what condition, and the use of tried and tested techniques, you can become a more accomplished taper. Bunch *et al.*[39] stated that tape becomes ineffective primarily due to the taper's inexperience. Well, nobody is born knowing how to tape, but if you know and understand the functional anatomy of the region to be taped you are a long way down the road to becoming a good taper; the rest is down to guidance, practice and experience.

- **Knowing the capabilities and limitations of tape in supporting an injury and in the prophylaxis of injury occurrence**

  Plaster of Paris, will, to all intents and purposes, stop all ranges of joint motion and protect an area that has been severely damaged (a fracture, for example). Braces range from extreme support to something that is tantamount to wearing a sock or sleeve. Likewise, tape can be very restrictive or allow for greater mobility while protecting an injury site. It is up to the taper to decide how much support is needed, especially if the person has never been taped before. It may be that you will want to consider input from the individual being taped (how tight or loose, for example), especially if they are taped on a regular basis. However, you should be realistic in your expectation of what tape can achieve, and inform the individual being taped of your thoughts. Bear in mind to remain positive as the "participants perceptions may contribute to its (tape) effectiveness in injury prevention"[40,41]. The question of whether or not tape is prophylactic is not a simple yes or no answer. How protective tape will be will depend on several factors:

- The individual's biomechanics

- Proprioception

- Neuromotor control
- Previous injury
- Extent of current injury and phase of recovery
- Effective application of tape.

In athletes there are other aspects to take into account, such as:

- The individual's skill level
- The terrain (used in the sport or activity)
- Equipment used e.g. the effect of leverage that a tennis racket could have on a wrist injury
- The extent of tackling or being tackled
- Speed, duration, direction and repetition of forces placed on the injury site
- The patient's activities of daily living and work.

Having said this, there is ample evidence that tape does play a prophylactic role[2-7].

TIP:

It is a good idea to have a personal checklist prior to taping to make sure you have not forgotten anything. For example:

- You must have a diagnosis
- You must know the mechanism of injury and repair
- You must never tape instead of treatment
- You can use as part of a rehabilitation programme
- You must know the rules of the sport (what you can and can't use)
- You must know what the athlete's needs / wants are (amount of support / comfort)
- You must have appropriate tape(s)
- You NEVER tape for no reason

REFERENCES

1. Frett TA, Reilly, TJ. Athletic taping. In: Mellion MB (ed) Sports medicine secrets: Philadelphia: Hanley and Belfus, 1994: 339–342.

2. Verhagen EA, Van Mechelen W, de Vente W. The effects of preventative measures on the incidence of ankle sprains. Clin J Sports Med 2000; 10: 291–296.

3. Ricard MD, Sherwood SM, Schulthies SS et al. Effects of tape on dynamic ankle inversion. J Athl Train 2000; 35: 31–37.

4. Olmstead LC, Vela LI, Deneger CR et al. Prophylactic ankle taping and bracing: a numbers needed to treat and cost benefit analysis. J Athl Train 2004; 39: 95–100.

5. Vicenzino B, Franettovich M, McPoil T et al. The effects of anti pronation tape on medial longitudinal arch during walking and running. Br J Sports Med 2005; 39: 939–943.

6. Moiler K, Hall T, Robinson K. The role of fibular tape in the prevention of ankle injury in basketball: a pilot study. J Orthop Sports Phys Ther 2006; 36: 661–668.

7. Ivins D. Acute ankle sprains: an update. Am Fam Physician 2006; 10: 1714–1720.

8. Lohrer H, Alt W, Gollhofer A. Neuromuscular properties and functional aspects of taped ankles. Am J Sports Med 1999; 27: 69–75.

9. Alt W, Lohrer H, Gollhofer A. Functional properties of adhesive ankle taping: neuromuscular and mechanical effects before and after exercise. Foot Ankle Int 1999; 20: 238–245.

10. Wilkerson GB. Biomechanical and neuromuscular effects of ankle taping and bracing. J Athl Train 2002; 37: 436–445.

11. Shima N, Maeda A, Hirohashi K. Delayed latency of peroneal reflex to sudden inversion with ankle taping and bracing. Int J Sports Med 2005; 26: 476–480.

12. Alexander CM, McMullan M, Harrison PJ. What is the effect of taping along or across a muscle on motorneurone excitability? A study using triceps surae. Man Ther 2008; 13(1): 57–62.

13. Kilbreath SL, Perkins S, Crosbie J et al. Gluteal taping improves hip extension during stance phase of walking following stroke. Aust J Physiother 2006; 52: 53–56.

14. Callaghan MJ, Selfe J, Bagley PJ et al. The effects of patella taping on knee joint propriocepction. J Athl Train 2002; 37: 19–24.

15. Callaghan MJ, Self J, McHenry A et al. Effects of patella taping on knee joint proprioception in patients with patellofemoral pain syndrome. Man Ther 2008; 13: 192–199.

16. Refshauge KM, Kilobreath SL, Raymond J. The effects of recurrent ankle inversion sprain and taping on proprioception at the ankle. Med Sci Sports Exerc 2000; 32: 10–15.

17. Robbins S, Waked E, Rappel R. Ankle taping improves proprioception before and after exercise in young men. Br J Sports Med 1995; 29: 242–247.

18. Leanderson J, Ekstam S, Salomonsson C. Taping of the ankle – the effect on postural sway during perturbation, before and after a training session. Knee Surg Sports Traumatol Arthrosc 1996; 4: 53–56.

19. Sinoneau GG, Degner RM, Kramper CA et al. Changes in ankle joint proprioception resulting from strips of athletic tape applied over the skin. J Athl Train 1997; 32: 141–147.

20. Tropp, H. Functional ankle instability revisited. J Athl Train 2002; 37: 512–515.

21. Fong DT, Hong Y, Chan LK et al. A systematic review on ankle injury and ankle sprain in sport. Sports Med 2007; 37: 73–94.

22. Herrington L. The effect of corrective taping of the patella on patella position as defined by MRI. Res Sports Med 2006; 14: 215–223.

23. Simmonds JV, Keer JR. Hypermobility and the hypermobility syndrome. Man Ther 2007; 12: 298–309.

24. Viljakka T, Rokkanen P. The treatment of ankle sprain by bandaging and antiphlogistic drugs. Ann Chir Gynaecol 1983; 72: 66–70.

25. Van Dijk CN. CBO-guideline for diagnosis and treatment of the acute ankle injury. National Organization for Quality Assurance in Hospitals. Ned Tijdschr Geneeskd 1999; 143: 2097–2101.

26. McConnell J. A novel approach to pain relief pre-therapeutic exercise. J Sci Med Sport 2000; 3: 325–334.

27. Kofotolis ND, Kellis E, Vlachopoulos SP. Ankle sprain injuries and risk factors in amateur soccer players during a 2 year period. Am J Sports Med 2007; 35(3): 458–466.

28. Emery CA, Meeuwisse WH, McAllister JR. Survey of sports participation and sports injury in Calgary and area high schools. Clin J Sports Med 2006; 16: 20–26.

29. Purdam CR, Fricker PA, Cooper B. Principles of treatment and rehabilitation. In: Bloomfield J, Fricker PA, Fitch KD (eds) Science and medicine in sport. Oxford: Blackwell Science, 1995: 246–263.

30. Oakes BW. Tendon-ligament basic science. In: Harries M, Williams C, Stanish WD et al (eds) Oxford textbook of sports medicine. Oxford: Oxford University Press, 1996: 493–511.

31. Torres JL. Ankle sprains. In: Brown DE, Neumann RD (eds) Orthopedic secrets. Philadelphia: Hanley and Belfus, 1995: 323–327.

32. Zainuddin Z, Hope P, Newton M et al. Effects of partial immobilization after eccentric exercise on recovery from muscle damage. J Athl Train 2005; 40: 197–202.

33. Eckstein F, Hudelmaier M, Putz R. The effects of exercise on human articular cartilage. J Anat 2006; 208: 491–512.

34. Urso ML, Scrimgeour AG, Chen YW et al. Analysis of human skeletal muscle after 48h immobilisation reveals alterations in mRNA and protein for extracellular matrix components. J Appl Physiol 2006; 101: 1136–1148.

35. Hudelmaier M, Glaser C, Hausschild A et al. Effects of joint unloading and reloading on human cartilage morphology and function, muscle cross-sectional areas, and bone density a quantitative case report. J Musculoskelet Neuronal Interact 2006; 6: 284–290.

36. Watson T. Tissue healing. Electrotherapy on the web. Available online at: www.electrotherapy.org.

37. Lederman E. Assisting repair with manual therapy. In: The science and practice of manual therapy. Edinburgh: Elsevier, 2005: 13–30.

38. Hardy MA. The biology of scar tissue formation. Phys Ther 1989; 69: 1014–1024.

39. Bunch RP, Bednarski K, Holland D et al. Ankle joint support: a comparison of reusable lace on brace with tapping and wrapping. Phys Sports Med 1985; 13: 59–62.

40. Sawkins K, Refshauge K, Kilbreath S et al. The placebo effect on taping in ankle instability. Med Sci Sport Exerc 2007; 39: 781–787.

41. Hunt E, Short S. Collegiate athletes' perceptions of adhesive ankle taping: a qualitative analysis. J Sports Rehab 2006; 15(4).

Section 1

PRINCIPLES

Chapter 1 TAPING SUPPLIES

Any successful taping job begins with choosing quality materials. Top-quality tape is more reliable and consistent than poor-quality tape and is essential if optimal protection is to be achieved. Tape quality affects the degree of compression, stability and support necessary for a properly executed taping technique.

Included in this chapter are descriptions of and uses for various tapes and supplies. These have been divided into two lists. The recommended essentials for taping are included in the first list. The optional supplies in the second list should also be available but are not mandatory. Many more items could be added to a well-equipped taping kit but we have covered only what we deem to be the most important supplies.

RECOMMENDED SUPPLIES

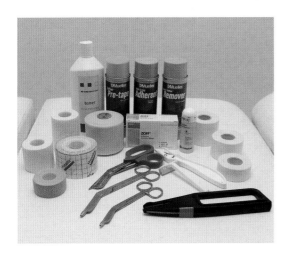

Essential taping supplies

- disposable razor and soap
- skin toughener spray
- quick-drying adhesive spray
- lubricating ointment/petroleum jelly (Vaseline™)
- heel and lace pads
- underwrap
- Comfeel™
- non-elastic (zinc oxide) tape 2.5 cm (1 in) and 5 cm (2 in) width. Wider tape useful in reinforcing vertical support strips
- elastic adhesive bandage 2.5 cm (1 in), 5 cm (2 in) and 7.5 cm (3 in) width
- fixation tape (Fixamol™, Sanipore™, Hyperfix™)
- bandage scissors
- padding: felt, foam or gel pad
- cohesive bandages 2.5 cm (1 in), 5 cm (2 in) and 7.5 cm (3 in) width

Additional items for field kit

- surgical gloves
- wound wash
- antiseptic solution
- Kaltostat™ (fibrous blood coagulant dressing)
- Tuff-cut shears
- cotton gauze squares: sterile and non-sterile
- plastic Band-Aid strips
- triangular bandages
- collar and cuff
- ice and towels
- pen, pencil and paper
- cellular/mobile phone

Optional supplies

- instant cold packs
- antifungal spray or powder
- blister protectors
- cotton-tipped applicators
- tongue depressors
- waterproof tape
- white zinc oxide tape 1.2 cm (½ in) width
- adhesive remover
- tape cutters
- nail clippers, nail scissors

ELASTIC ADHESIVE BANDAGE (EAB)

This tape offers elasticity as well as adhesion. Useful for a wide range of purposes:

- maintaining localized compression over a contusion
- keeping maximal pressure over an injury without compromising circulation
- forming an 'anchor' around a muscle area
- keeping a brace in place.

Quality characteristics

- strong recoil. To test, stretch an 80 cm (32 in) strip to maximum length. Hold for 30 seconds, then release. Tape should return to 125% of original length (100 cm; 40 in)
- ideally the roll should be encased in airtight wrapping to maintain freshness

Inferior

- little, ineffective or no recoil
- tendency to unravel at the edges
- does not adhere well; tends to peel off easily

ANTISEPTIC LOTION; ANTIFUNGAL SPRAY OR POWDER

Useful as a secondary precaution in treating minor abrasions, blisters, lacerations and tape cuts.

- apply to cleaned wounds prior to taping
- use sparingly so as not to interfere with the adhesive properties of the overall tape job

NON-ELASTIC (ZINC OXIDE) TAPE

The basic all-purpose tape essential to any taping kit used in any sport. Adhesive, non-elastic and available in rolls of various lengths, zinc oxide tape is indispensable for the athletic taper.

Quality characteristics

- slightly porous to permit some lateral glide or stretch (shearing) across the bias of the tape
- to test: grasp a 5 cm (2 in) piece of tape between your two hands and pull laterally. The tape should shear about 20° in either direction without creasing (as in the photographs below)

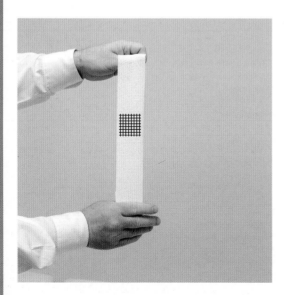
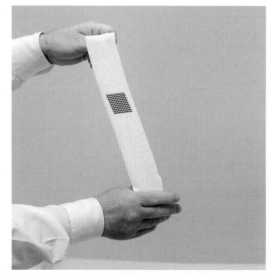
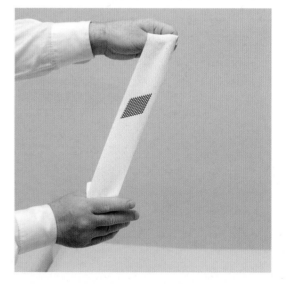

Inferior

- when tested as described above, a poor grade of tape will start to crease and to stick together almost as soon as any sideways stress is induced. Other types of inexpensive tape may have two or more lengths stitched end to end. Although the quality may not be inferior, it will not give a smooth, uniform finish to the taping job (important when the athlete is wearing footwear). Any seams must be removed before applying the tape

FIXATION TAPE (FIXAMOL™, SANIPORE™, HYPERFIX™)

This tape is primarily promoted for holding dressings in place. However, it also makes an excellent anchor when combined with adhesive spray, especially when encircling the whole limb is impractical or contraindicated; in such cases it can be used instead of non-elastic zinc oxide tape or elastic adhesive bandage. For many tapers, it is the tape of choice as an anchor in unloading (of neural/fascial elements for pain relief) techniques.

Quality characteristics

- strong
- hypoallergenic adhesive
- highly adhesive
- highly porous (allows skin to breathe)

Inferior

- can be awkward to use in long strips
- if it adheres to itself you cannot separate it

SKIN TOUGHENER SPRAY

Fast-drying aerosol spray that forms a thin adhesive layer protecting skin from contact with tape irritants and provides additional adhesive potency.

Quality characteristics

- dries quickly
- adheres well

Inferior

- can irritate sensitive skin
- difficult to remove

NOTE:

All types of tape should be kept in a cool, dry place. Rotate supplies to ensure freshness: old tape gets too sticky and difficult to use.

TIP:

Some brands are less apt to cause irritation in specific chemical-sensitive athletes. Having several brands on hand will enable the taper to try alternatives with different chemical ingredients.

ADHESIVE SPRAY

Quick-drying adhesive sprays applied directly to the skin help to keep tape from slipping.

Quality characteristics

- dries quickly
- adheres well

Inferior

- irritates skin
- difficult to remove

UNDERWRAP

Applied to the taping area between 'anchors', this thin foam material reduces the area of direct skin contact, protects skin from traction burns and tape irritation (zinc oxide and adhesive elements in tape are frequently the cause of skin irritations or allergic reactions).

The use of underwrap can be helpful when taping bony areas which are particularly susceptible to skin blisters and tape cuts.

Quality characteristics

- very fine-grained, thin foam roll that is slightly stretchy but non-adhesive. Normal width 5 cm (2 in)
- available in a wide range of colours as well as skintone

Inferior

- too thin – tears easily, tends to roll at edges producing irritating ridges if pulled over contours
- too thick – reduces efficacy of tape, not cost efficient since length of roll is significantly less as width increases

COMFEEL™ (COLOPLAST™)

A fast-drying liquid that forms a protective film ('second skin'). This product can be expensive if you are working to a budget.

Quality characteristics

- very easy to apply
- protects the skin from irritation
- waterproof, elastic and semi-permeable

Inferior

- pungent aroma on application, should be used only in a well-ventilated space
- can be expensive

TIP:
Essential in difficult taping situations of high humidity or where immersion in water makes adhesiveness a problem, i.e. a swimmer returning to action.

NOTE:
May be interchanged with skin toughener spray in situations where adherence is the primary concern.

TIP:
When choosing underwrap, thinness is preferable. However, if the material is too thin, the edges tend to roll more easily, causing ridges.

LUBRICATING OINTMENT/PETROLIUM JELLY

Viscous lubricating ointments used to decrease friction between tape and skin. These can be used instead of heel and lace pads if necessary.

Quality characteristics

- maintains viscosity at body temperature
- petroleum based

Inferior

- thin, water based
- will not maintain viscosity at body temperature

HEEL AND LACE PADS

Thin foam squares used in areas where there is a likelihood of friction under the taping, such as at the laces of the anterior ankle and the heel (used with a layer of skin lubricant).

Quality characteristics

- thin but sturdy
- does not flake or break when bent
- smooth finish

Inferior

- rough surface
- easily torn or broken

STERILE GAUZE PADS

Pads with a non-stick surface are useful for open wounds. They are used to:

- cleanse abrasions and lacerations with antiseptic solution
- protect open areas after cleaning blisters, lacerations, minor cuts and abrasions.

Quality characteristics

- firmly woven
- individually wrapped

Inferior

- poorly packaged: unlikely to offer reliable sterility

TIP:
Care must be taken to apply only a minimal amount so that the stability and support of the entire tape job are not jeopardized.

NOTE:
Lubrication is essential when taping high-friction areas, e.g. the tendo Achilles insertion, and sensitive skin areas (e.g. the front of the ankle, which is underlaid with superficial tendons, making the skin prone to blisters and/or tape cuts).

TIP:
For economy, thin sheets of aerated plastic packing can be cut into 7 cm (2¾ in) squares. Gauze squares may also be used.

NOTE:
Be careful when opening these pads: they must be sterile when applied to a wound.

Section 1: PRINCIPLES

NON-STERILE GAUZE PADS

These are used:

- to cleanse around abrasions and lacerations
- to apply pressure near a wound in order to arrest bleeding
- for splinting and protecting small areas such as a fractured toe.

Quality characteristics

- firmly woven

Inferior

- flimsy weave

ELASTIC BANDAGE/COHESIVE BANDAGE/ELASTIC WRAP

One of the most versatile components of a taping kit. It sticks to itself without sticking to skin or hair which means there is no need to shave the area and the taper may do away with underwrap for that reason. It is breathable, very durable and provides consistent compression.

A variety of different widths are available and the sizes most commonly used are:

- 15 cm (6 in): support for thigh and groin strains, splint supports, holding ice packs in place, compression on soft tissue injuries, temporarily wrapping other tape jobs while adhesive 'sets'
- 10 cm (4 in): support for ankle sprains, devising a makeshift sling, holding ice packs in place, compression on soft tissue injuries, temporarily wrapping other tape jobs while adhesive 'sets'
- 8 cm (3 in): small ankles, large wrists, compression on soft tissue injuries
- 5 cm (2 in): wrist sprains, children's injuries, compression on soft tissue injuries.

Quality characteristics

- firm weave
- good elasticity: should have a wide stretch with gradually increasing resistance
- good recoil: should return to within 10% of original length after use
- 'clingy' surface: reduces slippage between layers and holds position on limb

Inferior

- looser weave
- poor elasticity: stretches too easily and stops suddenly at limit of expansion
- poor recoil: tends to stay stretched after use; does not return to within 20% of original length after use
- too smooth a surface: tends to slip between layers and slides down limb

TIP:
There are a number of other applications where elastic bandages will prove useful. The well-appointed taping kit should have these bandages in a range of sizes and in sufficient quantity to handle diverse situations.

FOAM PADDING

Thin sheets made of dense foam, useful when taping a bruised area; for example, when taping a bruised tibia (shinbone), a layer of padding can help protect the injured area.

Quality characteristics

- 'closed cell' foam: offers good protection as it is firm in construction and waterproof

Inferior

- thick, spongy appearance

SURGICAL FELT PADDING

Sheets of densely compressed fibres, used as protection and support when taping a damaged acromio-clavicular joint shoulder, for example, or as temporary heel lifts supporting full body weight.

Quality characteristics

- firm, even texture
- soft to the touch
- equal thickness throughout sheet

Inferior

- too loosely woven to protect adequately or to provide support when subjected to continuous weight bearing
- if fibres are too tightly compressed, cutting is difficult and splitting impossible
- uneven thickness over the sheet

NOTE:
When effective taping requires local pressure and firm protection such as a separated shoulder, felt padding is preferable as it gives a more solid, cushioning effect than foam. Light and tightly compacted felt is used to make heel lifts.

TIP:
A thick sheet of quality felt can be split to make thinner layers.

GEL PADDING

Gel pads come in many forms: as a sock, sleeve or pad. Used for anti-shock, to reduce friction and to reduce problems caused by pressure and shearing forces.

Quality characteristics

- does not tear
- conforms to the body, especially around bony prominences
- washable and reusable

Inferior

- can be uncomfortable if too thick
- can be difficult to cut and shape if too thick

PLASTERS (COMPEED™, BAND-AID™)

Available in a variety of widths and lengths, useful for simple cuts and grazes. Some brands are waterproof.

Quality characteristics

- wrapped singly
- adheres well

Inferior

- may be non-sterile
- poor adherence

Inferior (fabric strips)

- poor adherence
- often stretch to the point of forming creases which may cause secondary blisters

TAPE CUTTERS

Often referred to as 'sharks' because of their shape.

- plastic handle encasing a replaceable razor sharp blade (take care when using or changing this blade as it is very sharp)
- flattened tip helps protect the skin when removing tape
- particularly helpful in removing ankle or wrist taping when scissoring action is awkward or impossible

TIP:
Tape cutters are useful when handling large numbers of ankle tapings and speed is critical.

BANDAGE SCISSORS

Special-purpose scissors with a flattened tip that protects the underlying skin from the cutting surface during tape removal.

CASE HISTORY FORMS

Keep an accurate record of past and present medical complaints (including musculo-skeletal) as well as current procedures.

Essential information includes:

- the patient's name, address, date of birth and contact phone numbers
- family physician's details
- site of injury (body part)
- date of injury
- full details of injury (consequence)
- current health and medical information
- past health and medical information

Recommended supplies

- medication
- full examination of injury and associated areas
- treatment administered (if any) and subsequent care suggested or implemented.

Additional information for athletes

- sports participated in
- level of participation
- how often do they train/compete
- intensity and amount of training
- type of training
- club details
- who else has input on this injury (coach, trainer, manager, surgeon, etc. so that you can liaise with them)

This information is vital for statistical records and it can also be crucial should medico-legal complications arise or if the treatment provided were to be challenged. The importance of keeping detailed records cannot be stressed too strongly.

SURGICAL GLOVES

Non-sterile, thin, disposable rubber gloves.

- mandatory when attending to any wound oozing blood or serum. Even though an abrasion or laceration may seem insignificant, blood carries transmissible infections
- for maximum protection, surgical gloves should be used when treating even minor injuries
- change gloves between patients to prevent cross-infection
- dispose of soiled gloves correctly

Quality characteristics

- thin yet strong
- stretch without tearing

Inferior

- prone to tearing and puncture easily
- when ultra-thin, afford little protection in instances where the skin is broken

CELLULAR/MOBILE PHONE

When a major injury requires ambulance transport or supplementary medical personnel, reaction time is critical. Having a cell/mobile phone or exact change for a payphone PLUS a list of emergency telephone numbers for the area will facilitate summoning emergency assistance.

NOTE:
When there is any doubt as to the reliability of a pair of surgical gloves, two pairs of gloves should be worn.

NOTE:
Thick, clumsy gloves hinder the dexterity necessary to produce an effective taping application.

Taping Supplies

OPTIONAL SUPPLIES

WHITE NON-ELASTIC ZINC OXIDE TAPE

Narrow tape 1.2 cm (½ in) useful in taping small joints such as toes, fingers and thumbs.

ADHESIVE REMOVER

Dissolves adhesive and removes adhesive residue.

- helpful when tape has been left on for longer than 24 hours
- skin must be washed thoroughly after using tape remover to avoid irritation

TONGUE DEPRESSOR/FLAT WOODEN STICKS

Apart from the obvious use, these are useful when applying lubricants or ointments to stop hands becoming oily or greasy.

COTTON BUDS

Preferable to cotton pads for precise application of gels, creams, oil or when applying skin toughener or adhesive spray near eyes or open wounds.

BLISTER PROTECTION (SECOND SKIN™ OR COMPEED™)

- essential in the treatment of blisters
- allows patients to remain active while protecting the area from exacerbation

TRIANGULAR BANDAGE, COLLAR AND CUFF, MUSLIN SQUARES

Useful as a binding or as a strap for splints.

- can be used as a sling for arm/shoulder injuries
- provide padding and/or compression

WATERPROOF TAPE

- essential in humid weather or water-related events
- effective as a waterproof covering for other tape applications

NAIL CLIPPERS, NAIL SCISSORS

Useful for removing ripped nails or for trimming prior to taping.

NOTE:
Avoid spraying chemicals near eyes or open wounds as this can be dangerous.

TIP:
If blister protection is applied to vulnerable areas prior to participation, blisters are less likely to develop.

The rationale for taping is to provide protection and support for an injured part while permitting optimal functional movement. An essential rehabilitation tool, taping enhances healing by allowing early activity within carefully controlled ranges that can facilitate a faster recovery from injury.[1-7] Taping also permits an earlier return to activity, play or competition by protecting the area from further injury or exacerbation of the existing injury and avoiding compensatory injuries elsewhere such as delayed hip muscle activation, as can happen with severe ankle injuries.[8] Taping also reduces pain (for a full explanation, see the Epilogue).

TAPE VERSUS BRACE

There is ample evidence to suggest that in many cases the use of a brace is as good as and in some cases more efficient than tape at supporting and promoting the repair of damaged tissues.[9-23] However, certain types of braces are inappropriate (usually those with metal, hard plastic or carbon fibre), especially in contact sports. Tape is usually the support of choice, especially when the athlete can return to activity, training and competition with the assistance of the support that tape can offer.

We have to ask the question: if an athlete needs significant support in order to train or compete, should they be doing it? The answer of course is **NO**! Likewise, if after taping the individual still experiences pain with activity, they should **STOP**! The tape should be removed and the injury should be reevaluated.

BRACING

- No expertise needed; can be applied by the patient
- Reusable
- Non-allergenic
- Adjustable
- Cost-effective
- Certain braces may be banned from some sports

TAPING

- Individually applied
- Less bulky than a brace
- Caters for unusual anatomy
- Some expertise needed to apply
- Acceptable form of support in all sports

2

PURPOSES AND BENEFITS

The purposes and benefits of correctly applied tape jobs are delineated as follows.

PURPOSES

- Supports an injured structure
- Limits harmful ranges of motion
- Enhances repair and recovery
- Allows pain-free functional movement
- Permits protected resumption of activities
- Decreases pain

BENEFITS

- Circulation is enhanced through pain-free movement
- Swelling is controlled
- Prevents:
  a. worsening of initial injury
  b. compensatory injury to adjacent parts
  c. atrophy from non-use

- Allows:
  a. continued body conditioning and strength often lost during postinjury inactivity
  b. maintenance of ability to react often lost due to inhibitive factors (pain, fear of reinjury)

HOW LONG CAN YOU LEAVE TAPE ON FOR?

Sports tape is designed to stay on for the duration of the sport and then it should be removed. Care must be taken when taping, especially when encircling an area of the body as the blood and nerve supplies can be compromised (see below). Always get feedback from the individual, check for signs of a compromised blood supply and ask appropriate questions for a compromised nerve supply. When support is needed for longer periods, one should select the appropriate materials and techniques and warn the individual of what to be aware of and to remove the tape and seek advice if they are unsure.

Taping can only be truly beneficial if the injury is properly assessed and diagnosed and the appropriate taping technique is utilized. An inappropriate taping technique can place strain on associated regions, cause blisters or irritation and, in some cases, increase the severity of the injury and cause further damage to surrounding structures.

In order to apply the tape safely and effectively, it is essential that the taper appreciate both the aims of taping and situations to avoid. In this chapter, these criteria are outlined.

PRETAPING CONSIDERATIONS

Always explain the reasons for taping to the patient so that they are fully informed of why you are recommending tape and they can give their consent to be taped. Always enquire if they have experienced allergic reactions to tape. A simple question is usually sufficient, such as 'Is your skin irritated by wearing a Band-Aid?'. If in doubt, you may apply a small test patch of tape to the skin as a method of assessment. If the patient does have known allergic reactions or develops one, try underwrap or hypoallergenic tapes or skin balms. **Should the patient feel any irritation from the tape at any time, it should be removed immediately and the skin washed and cleaned**.

By using the mnemonic **S.U.P.P.O.R.T.** to review the goals of effective taping, the taper can quickly run through a critical checklist before choosing the best technique and materials for that particular injury.

NOTE:

Taping alone is not a definitive treatment: for your convenience, charts have been included in Chapter Four (Basic Pathology) and Chapters Six to Nine (Techniques) to help put the taping in perspective relative to the entire treatment plan.

S SWELLING must be controlled by adequate padding and/or compression to prevent irritating exudates and other fluids from accumulating (oedema) and to ensure the best environment for tissue regeneration and repair.

U UNDUE STRESS to the injured region must be prevented so as to reduce the possibility of additional injury or of increasing the severity of the injury.

P PROTECTION of the area from further soft tissue damage (i.e. bruises, blisters, tape cuts) by using pads, lubricants and other protective materials.

P PAIN and discomfort must be minimized by supporting the injured part, by controlling unnecessary or excessive movement, and by taking care not to cause further irritation to the injured tissues.

O OPTIMAL healing and tissue repair can be enhanced through correctly applying tape, keeping the range of motion within safe limits and maintaining continuous compression.

R REHABILITATION of the tissues to a fully functional state (joint mobility, soft tissue flexibility, muscle strength, ligament stability, neuromotor control and proprioception) must be considered when choosing the right taping technique adaptation for the appropriate stage of rehabilitation (subacute, functional, return to sport).

T THERAPEUTIC CARE in the early stages of treatment is critical for a rapid recovery. Treatment may include the application of electrical modalities (ultrasound, laser, interferential electrotherapy, muscle stimulation, etc.), manual treatment and exercise therapy to control pain and swelling and to promote rapid healing.

POSTTAPING CONSIDERATIONS

In addition to being aware of the purposes of a particular taping application, there are conditions or situations to observe or to avoid after the taping is completed. The mnemonic

P. R. E. C. A. U. T. I. O. N. will help you recall several important points after taping.

P PREMATURE participation in an activity which involves the injured part must be avoided. A major mistake many patients, especially athletes, make is returning to action too soon. This can delay healing and often results in reinjury to the weakened structures as well as increasing the chance of further complications to the compensatory areas.

R RANGE OF MOTION should be restricted but maintained as close as possible to normal for the body part involved. Severe limitation of motion can result in an overextension of surrounding or compensatory structures, prolong repair and recovery and lead to tissue changes in and around the joint injured.[24-27] Permitting too free a range of motion will not adequately protect the tissues involved and can leave them prone to further injury.

E EXPERT opinion must be obtained when any serious injury, particularly a fracture, dislocation or tissue rupture, is suspected. Also, a paying agency or government regulation may require a physician's assessment prior to treatment.

C CIRCULATION in the injured area must be monitored for any sign of constriction. Pressure bandages must be checked regularly.

A ALLERGIES AND SKIN IRRITATIONS present a very real problem, one that is frustrating for both the patient and the taper. The more serious degree of allergic reaction results in localized blistering, welts, pustules, rashes and pain. Simple irritation is generally a less severe reaction of reddened skin or small blisters.

U UNDUE DEPENDENCY ON TAPING is a psychological danger which may arise when patients, especially athletes, think that they cannot perform without taping. In such cases the injured area may not return to its preinjury performance level. Associated with prolonged immobility, this situation may lead to the patient spending unnecessary time having manual therapy to overcome the results of excessive or prolonged taping.

T TENDONS, MUSCLES AND BODY PROMINENCES must be treated with special care and attention so as to avoid pressure build-up and friction.

I ICE should **not** be applied to an injured part that is to be immediately subjected to taping. The temporary reduction of tissue volume due to icing will result in a taping that will tighten progressively as the body part warms up. Also, patients may have reduced skin sensation after icing, and tissue injury can result from such sensory loss.

O ONLY top-quality supplies should be used in order to ensure a consistently high standard of tape application.

N NERVE conduction and local sensation may be affected by secondary inflammation or by the taping job itself. It is essential to evaluate the level of sensation prior to taping so that factors altering sensation can be assessed properly.

REFERENCES

1. Kerhoffs GM, Rowe BH, Assendelft WJ et al. Immobilization for acute ankle sprain: a systemic review. Arch Orthop Trauma Surg 2001; 121: 462-471.

2. Kerhoffs GM, Rowe BH, Assendelft WJ et al. Immobilisation and functional treatment for acute lateral ankle ligament injuries in adults. Cochrane Database Syst Rev 2002;(3):CD003762.

3. Costa ML, Shepstone l, Darrah C et al. Immediate full-weight-bearing mobilization for repaired Achilles tendon ruptures: a pilot study. Injury 2003; 34: 874-876.

4. Costa ML, MacMillan K, Halliday D et al. Randomised controlled trials of immediate weight-bearing mobilisation for rupture of the tendo Achillis. J Bone Joint Surg Br 2006; 88: 69-77.

5. Feiler S. Taping like in professional sports: targeted stabilization and early mobilization of the ankle. Fortschritte de Medizin 2006; 148: 47-49.

6. Jacob KM, Paterson R. Surgical repair followed by functional rehabilitation for acute and chronic achilles tendon injuries: excellent functional results, patient satisfaction and no re-ruptures. Aust NZ J Surg 2007; 77: 287-291.

7. Maripuri SN, Debnath UK, Rao P, Mohanty K. Simple elbow dislocation among adults: a comparative study of two different methods of treatment. Injury 2007; 38(11): 1254-1258.

8. Bullock-Saxton JE, Janda V, Bullock MI. The influence of ankle sprain injury on muscle activation during hip extension. Int J Sports Med 1994; 15: 330-334.

9. Burks RT, Bean BG, Marcus R, Barker HB. Analysis of athletic performance with prophylactic ankle devices. Am J Sports Med 1991; 19: 104-106.

10. Paris DL. The effects of the Swede-O, new cross, and McDavid ankle braces and adhesive taping on speed, balance, agility, and vertical jump. J Athl Train 1992; 27: 253-256.

11. Paris DL, Kokkaliaris J, Vardaxis V. Ankle ranges of motion during extended activity periods while taped and braced. J Athl Train 1995; 30: 223-228.

12. Verbrugge JD. The effects of semirigid Air-Stirrup bracing vs adhesive ankle taping on motor performance. J Orthop Sports Phys Ther 1996; 23: 320-325.

13. Jerosch J, Thorwesten L, Bork H et al. Is prophylactic bracing cost effective? Orthopaedics 1996; 19: 405-414.

14. Metcalf RC, Schlabach GA, Looney MA et al. A comparison of moleskin tape, linen tape and lace-up brace on joint restriction and movement performance. J Athl Train 1997; 32: 136-140.

15. Callaghan MJ. Role of ankle bracing and taping in the athlete. Br J Sports Med 1997; 31: 102-108.

16. Hume PA, Gerrard DF. Effectiveness of external ankle support. Bracing and taping in rugby union. Sports Med 1998; 25: 285-312.

17. Cordova ML, Ingersoll CD, LeBlanc MJ. Influence of ankle support on joint range of motion before and after exercise: a meta-analysis. Orthop Sports Phys Ther 2000; 30: 170-177.

18. Verhagen EA, van Mechelen W, de Vente W. The effect of preventative measures in the incidence of ankle sprains. Clin J Sports Med 2000; 10: 291-296.

19. Handoll HH, Rowe BH, Quinn KM et al. Interventions for preventing ankle ligament injuries. Cochran Database Sys Rev 2001; 3.

20. Barkoukis V, Sykaras E, Costa F et al. Effectiveness of taping and bracing in balance. Percept Mot Skills 2002; 94: 566-574.

21. Arnold BL, Docherty CL. Bracing and rehabilitation – what's new? Clin J Sports Med 2004; 23: 83-95.

22. Olmsted LC, Vela LI, Denegar CR et al. Prophylactic ankle taping and bracing: a numbers needed to treat and cost benefit analysis. J Athl Train 2004; 39: 95-100.

23. Boyce SH, Quigley MA, Campbell S. Management of ankle sprains: a randomised controlled trial of the treatment of inversion injuries using an elastic support bandage or an aicast brace. Br J Sports Med 2005; 39: 91-96.

24. Zainuddin Z, Hope P, Newton M et al. Effects of partial immobilization after eccentric exercise on recovery from muscle damage. J Athl Train 2005; 40: 197-202.

25. Eckstein F, Hudelmaier M, Putz R. The effects of exercise on human articular cartilage. J Anat 2006; 208: 491-512.

26. Urso ML, Scrimgeour AG, Chen YW et al. Analysis of human skeletal muscle after 48h immobilisation reveals alterations in mRNA and protein for extracellular matrix components. J Appl Physiol 2006; 101: 1136-1148.

27. Hudelmaier M, Glaser C, Hausschild A et al. Effects of joint unloading and reloading on human cartilage morphology and function, muscle cross-sectional areas, and bone density – a quantitative case report. J Musculoskelet Neuronal Interact 2006; 6(3): 284-290.

The choice of taping technique requires specific knowledge and observation skills. The following points are essential to ensure an effective, efficient taping application:

- a thorough knowledge of the anatomy of the area to be taped
- evaluation skills to assess:
  - a. structure(s) injured
  - b. degree of injury
  - c. stage of healing
- appropriate tape and choice of technique
- consideration of sport-specific needs (if applicable)
- be prepared to adapt your technique to suit individual needs
- adequate preparation of the area to be taped
- effective application of tape
- testing on completion of taping.

Deciding when to tape an injury, what techniques to apply for maximum effectiveness and how to test a completed job may seem a daunting task to the novice. To simplify and facilitate the process, three major stages of taping application with useful checklists follow. These will help the taper to quickly assess all the important factors critical to each stage. These stages are:

- PREAPPLICATION
- APPLICATION
- POSTAPPLICATION

Using the following outline as a guide, specific checklists for a particular sport or event may be devised with the assistance of someone who is familiar with the unique requirements of the sport/event and athletes involved therein.

PREAPPLICATION CHECKLIST

PRACTICAL: IS TAPING GOING TO WORK FOR THIS INJURY?

- Will tape adhere effectively to the body part?
- Does the area need to be prepared, e.g. cleaned and shaved?
- Is the athlete's skin damp or excessively oily?
- Are environmental factors likely to make taping impractical (weather or sport factors, i.e. rain, cold temperatures, high humidity; diving or swimming injury)?
- An athlete should not leave the treatment room with a taping job that does not stick; their false sense of security could lead to further injury.

LOGICAL: IS TAPING THE CORRECT PROCEDURE?

- Has the injury been adequately assessed and properly diagnosed? If you do not have the appropriate assessment skills, ensure that someone who does evaluates the athlete: which structures are injured, degree of injury, stage of healing?
- Is it possible that the athlete has an unhealed fracture, an unreduced dislocation or subluxation, etc. which would require medical attention? If so, taping would not be the appropriate intervention.
- In cases of concussion, profuse bleeding, abrasion, laceration, etc. **IMMEDIATE FIRST AID** and a trip to the emergency room are the treatments of choice – not taping.
- MATERIALS: WHAT IS NEEDED?

A quick review of the type and quantity of taping materials needed for the specific injury will facilitate a swift, organized taping job. Having the materials ready and within reach will maximize efficiency.

ASSESSMENT: WHAT IS INJURED OR AT RISK?

The ability to assess which body structures are injured (or at risk, either directly or indirectly), and to what degree, is essential in selecting the right taping application. A thorough knowledge of anatomy coupled with an understanding of the demands and requirements of specific sports are also essential elements in determining the appropriate taping technique. If tape is to be used as part of a rehabilitation regime, tapers will also need knowledge of the repair mechanism and stages of repair as they apply to the injured tissues, to enable them to select appropriate taping techniques. Application of this knowledge will become second nature through experience.

NOTE:
Should an athlete continue to participate in their sport with an incorrectly diagnosed injury, serious tissue damage could be the result and lead to a more complicated recovery process.

TIP:
A first aid course is highly recommended and in many cases is mandatory when involved in the treatment of sports-related injuries.

TIP:
Practising on simulated injuries helps improve decision-making and taping skills.

*The following general points should be considered **before** taping an injury.*

JOINT RANGE AND MUSCLE FLEXIBILITY: WHAT IS THE ATHLETE'S NORM?

Although this range differs from athlete to athlete, testing and examination of the corresponding uninjured joint and muscle area should be helpful in delineating these factors. This procedure will also ensure that the taping will not excessively limit the range of motion of the injured area.

PROBLEM AREAS: SUPERFICIAL SKIN DAMAGE IN CREASES OR BONY AREAS

Soft skin (in elbow or knee creases) and areas where tape pulls around bony points (the back of the heel in ankle taping) are often the sites of superficial skin damage.

Constant pressure from a poor tape job can cause painful pressure points (such as the styloid process at the base of the fifth metatarsal bone when an ankle is taped too tightly).

Arteries, veins, nerves or bones that are anatomically superficial (close to the skin surface) require extra care to avoid skin damage.

Trouble spots for each injury area should be reviewed before taping is attempted.

SPORT-SPECIFIC ITEMS: MEETING MOVEMENT DEMANDS OF THE ATHLETE

What is the range of motion required for the injured athlete's sport? For example, for a lateral ankle sprain, when taping a basketball player, the taping need is near-maximum plantarflexion (for jumping); in taping an ice hockey player, the requirement shifts to near-maximum dorsiflexion. In both cases the taping purpose is to prevent abnormal lateral mobility, yet the taping procedures must be different in order to accommodate the demands of a sport-specific range of motion. Even within a sport, there may be differences; for example, in rugby the needs of a forward player may be different from that of a back player. Don't be afraid to ask the athlete what they want or usually have done when taping. Very often, they will know what works for them and what they are comfortable with. Remember, whatever you do, it must be effective.

THE STARTING POSITION OF THE INJURED PART IN PREPARATION FOR TAPING

The best position is one in which the injured structure is unstressed (or neutral) and well supported (not stretched). Check that the athlete is sufficiently comfortable to maintain the required position throughout the taping procedure. The taper should also be able to work from an efficient, comfortable, biomechanically sound position.

APPLICATION CHECKLIST

PREPARATION OF THE INJURED AREA: SKIN CONDITION

- DIRTY: clean gently with a liquid antiseptic soap or antiseptic-soaked gauze. Pat dry. If skin is lacerated or abraded, apply a light layer of antibiotic ointment locally and cover with protective gauze. Always wear protective gloves when dealing with lacerations and abrasions.

- WET: dry gently with gauze. Use adhesive spray.

- OILY: wipe with rubbing alcohol-soaked gauze. Apply adhesive spray to ensure tape adhesion.

- HAIRY: shave area to be taped. Apply antiseptic lotion. Swab dry with gauze. Use a skin toughener if skin is not irritated.

- IRRITATED: apply a small amount of antibiotic ointment. Apply lubricant sparingly and use protective padding over the area.

CHOOSING THE CORRECT TAPE FOR A SPECIFIC TAPING JOB

As stated in Chapter Two, choosing the right type of tape depends on the actual structure(s) involved and whether the taping job involves padding, support, restraint or compression.

In general, **ELASTIC** tape is used for **contractile** tissue injuries (i.e. muscles, tendons). Elastic tape is preferable in these instances because it gives stretch with support and a graduated resistance, yet limits full stretch of the muscle or tendon.

Because muscles must be allowed a certain amount of normal expansion during activity, elastic tape should be used as **anchors** when encircling muscle bulk is required. It should also be used for specific **compression** taping requiring localized pressure.

NON-ELASTIC tape is used to support injuries of **non-contractile** structures (i.e. ligaments). Non-elastic tape reinforces the joints in the same way the ligaments would, thereby increasing joint stability.

TAPE APPLICATION

The person applying tape to an injury must modify the application to suit the circumstances specific to each situation, and the needs of each patient. Education and experience will enable the taper to develop variations on the basic techniques offered in this guide. Several ankle taping variations are illustrated in Chapter Six.

As long as the tape application is fulfilling the goal of supporting or protecting the targeted area without putting other structures at risk, a procedural variation can be used.

TIP:

In all taping procedures, protective layers with a lubricant should be used in areas particularly susceptible to irritation from taping, such as the back of the heel, Achilles tendon, anterior ankle, hamstring tendons, etc.

Section 1: PRINCIPLES

TAPING TECHNIQUES

The two main techniques used in applying tape are commonly referred to as strip taping and smooth roll.

Strip taping employs one short strip of tape at a time, in very specific directions and with highly controlled tension. This technique is often used in basic preventive taping as demonstrated in Chapter Six.

Smooth roll refers to use of a single, continuous, uninterrupted winding of a piece of tape.

	ADVANTAGES	DISADVANTAGES
Strip	• Accurate tension • Tape applied only where needed	• Requires time and practice
Smooth roll	• Quick to apply • Useful when taping an entire team	• Difficult to control tension accurately. • Tendency to use too much tape

NOTE:

The strip technique is demonstrated in this guide as we believe this to be more effective as it provides very specific localized support for the injured structures.

QUALITY CONTROL: WHILE THE TAPING IS IN PROGRESS, MONITOR THESE POINTS

- Is effective compression being maintained without loss of circulation?
- Is the tape adhering properly?
- Is the injured structure being properly supported by the technique chosen?
- Are the supporting strips and anchor points adequately tight?

POSTAPPLICATION CHECKLIST

MONITORING THE RESULTS: IS THE TAPING EFFECTIVE?

Follow these steps only when the tape job has been completed.

- Gently manually stress the joint movement to check for adequate limitation at the extremes of range of motion and in the direction of the injury.
- Check for stability of the joint and taping strips. The athlete should experience no pain during these tests.
- Further testing of the finished taping procedure involves functional tests in sport-specific movements as well as action and/or ranges of motion.
- Don't forget to ask the athlete 'Is it comfortable? Can you function adequately?'.

FUNCTIONAL TESTING: CAN THE ATHLETE SAFELY ENGAGE IN SPORT?

Before the athlete can return to training or competition, it is necessary to thoroughly evaluate the taping relative to performance of sport-specific skills and movements. These tests, performed in order of increasing difficulty and stress to the joints, should also be assessed by the medical support personnel.

Example of functional testing

Sport: Soccer

Injured area: Ankle

Testing progression:

- simple walking to jogging
- jogging on the spot
- running in a straight line
- running in a loose 'S' line
- running in a tight 'S' line
- running in a figure of eight
- cutting side to side at a jog (zig zags)
- cutting side to side at a run
- running backwards
- finally, jumping

NOTE:

At this point in testing, any ineffective taping should either be adjusted, to correct the problem that is causing the pain or loss of agility, or completely reapplied. The injury should be reassessed for the appropriateness of taping.

The last activity will test the athlete's ability to perform full-impact weight bearing on the ankle from a height – a position which places the ankle at its highest risk of reinjury.

If at any juncture in these tests the athlete experiences pain or loss of agility, the evaluation should be **STOPPED** before they suffer further injury or reinjury.

The key factors in determining whether or not the athlete can return to training and competition with the aid of tape are:

- monitoring ability and speed in sport-specific skills
- pain-free functional testing
- pain-free function on returning to training/competition.

TAPE REMOVAL

When the tape is no longer required, removal must be undertaken with the utmost care. The 'rip it off quick' approach should be avoided as it has the very real possibility of damaging the skin, creating a new injury and jeopardizing recovery.

Only appropriate bandage scissors or tape cutters (tape shark) should be used to avoid damage to the skin or other sensitive structures in the area.

The preferred method is to first select an area of soft tissue away from bone or bony prominences as these can be quite painful to cut across. Cut the tape using the blunt tip of the scissors and ease the skin away from the tape, forming a tunnel to facilitate cutting. After cutting the tape, carefully peel off slowly and gently, while pressing down on the exposed skin and pulling the tape back along itself, parallel (not perpendicular!) to the surface of the skin – keep it **low and slow**.

The safe removal of tape is demonstrated in the accompanying DVD.

ARE THERE ANY SIGNS OF SKIN IRRITATION OR BREAKDOWN?

Inspect the skin closely for signs of irritation, blisters, allergic reactions or any other adverse effects of the tape.

TIP:
A small amount of lubricant on the tip of the cutting instrument will help it glide underneath the tape.

The majority of injuries incurred during participation in sports activities are sprains, strains and contusions involving the musculo-skeletal system. The taping techniques demonstrated in this guide are particularly helpful for these conditions. Although some form of splinting and protection is also necessary for fractures, dislocations, nerve injuries, lacerations, abrasions and blisters, these conditions are beyond the intended scope of this guide.

In order to choose the appropriate tape and technique, you should first have a working knowledge of the repair process as it applies to the soft tissues. There are three recognized phases of healing.

1. **The acute phase**. This is the phase immediately following an injury which consists of an inflammatory process, to a greater or lesser degree, depending on the extent of the injury. During this phase, which lasts between 3 and 7 days,[1,2] taping is aimed at compressing the injury site. This means that a stretch tape such as a cohesive bandage would be the tape of choice, or a Tubigrip. These will compress the site while allowing movement when the tissues swell. Care should be taken not to apply the bandage or Tubigrip too tightly and the patient should be advised to remove any bandaging that is too tight and seek immediate advice.

2. **The proliferative phase**, so called due to the proliferation of cells during this phase. This is also known as the regeneration or matrix phase, as this is when a loose matrix is laid down to effect a temporary repair to the tissues. This is the phase when tape is applied so that the tissues can be stressed without causing further damage. So we would opt for a stronger taping technique during this phase. The loose matrix is easily damaged but the tissues need to be stressed in order for them to form a strong matrix along the lines of force.

3. **The remodelling phase** is, as the name suggests, the phase in which the tissues reform to 'normal'. No one at present knows when this phase is completed, as the cells of tissue repair have been found in and around an injury site up to 12 months after it was deemed that the injury had recovered.[3] During this phase we would opt for taping techniques that allow greater movement while still offering support.

Tape is reported to lose 20–40% of its effectiveness by approximately 20 minutes after application.[4,5] However, this does depend on the type of tape used.[6] This is a very negative way of reporting statistics and if we look at these from another perspective, we could say that tape retains 60–80% of its effectiveness after 20 minutes. However, joint control is increased when muscles are warm and therefore, the stabilizing effect of tape is more important during the initial stages of training or competition,[7] so we really only need tape to be maximally effective during this time.

We know that when athletes are fatigued there is a decrease in neuromotor control.[8] Tape may offer support that could have a prophylactic role when the athlete is fatigued.

R.I.C.E.S

Rest, Ice, Compression, Elevation, Support: this is a well-established protocol for initial first aid,[9-13] the evidence for which is largely anecdotal.[14,15] Regardless of this, it is one of the few aspects of treatment and rehabilitation that is agreed on by many therapists.[16-18] There are some questions you should ask of yourself before recommending R.I.C.E.S. to a patient.

- What does rest mean for this patient? Does it mean complete rest? Does it mean rest from those activities that are likely to exacerbate, maintain or create a new injury? If the answer to the second question is yes, then what activities can they do?

- The use of ice at present is controversial.[19-21] What do you expect from icing? Vasoconstriction? Vasodilation? Decreased pain? Does the site of the injury matter? Do superficial injuries need the same amount of icing time as deeper tissues? How long should you ice for and for what period of time?[18,19] Should you ice on the injury? Proximal to it? Or distal to it?

- The evidence for compressing an injury is at best ambiguous.[15,22,23] Many tapes, Tubigrips and braces will offer different levels of compression. Which one do you choose and why? Why do we compress the injury? How long do you need to compress the injury for? And for what period of time? How much compression is necessary?

- Many authors recommend elevating an injury. However, no evidence was found either for or against the use of such a treatment modality. How are you going to recommend that the patient elevate the injury site? Do they need to elevate a shoulder injury? How long should you elevate for and for what period of time?

- Support can take many guises; what type of support is going to be best for your patient?

STRUCTURES REQUIRING TAPING

The structures most often requiring taping are joints, ligaments, muscles, tendons and associated bony parts. The following brief description of these structures with specific taping considerations will help the beginner and serve as a review for the more advanced taper.

JOINTS

These are structures formed where two or more bones meet and move one on another. The movements of joints are controlled by ligaments, joint capsules, muscles, bone on bone and, of course, pathological factors. Friction is minimized by the smooth (hyaline) cartilage over the articulated surface of the bone and by the synovial fluid within the joint capsule of synovial joints.

Because of the complex interaction of muscles and tendons involved in joint movement, an injury to any link in the functional chain unbalances the entire structure; for example, a severe ankle injury can lead to compensatory misfiring of the hip muscles.[24] This imbalance causes pain and varying degrees of further joint dysfunction. Therefore, in taping joints, the primary concern is to support and protect the injured structure. Reestablishing the joint's delicate balance while optimizing mobility without shifting function and/or reliance to compensatory structures is also very important.

When a joint has been taped, the patient must go through specific functional movements to determine that joint balance has been restored and to evaluate compensatory stress. If the patient is an athlete then they should also perform sport-specific tasks. The patient should be able to perform all required motions without experiencing pain.

LIGAMENTS

These are non-elastic connective tissue structures that stabilize joints and reinforce joint capsules. When ligaments are stretched, torn or bruised, the resulting sprain requires careful taping in order to assist in establishing structural support and functional movement to the joint while preventing or reducing the threat of further injury to the ligament. Generally, a **non-elastic** taping application that appropriately restricts unwanted movement of the joint will allow the ligament to recover without further stress or trauma.

MUSCLE/TENDON UNITS

These are elastic contractile structures that produce movement of the musculo-skeletal system. An elastic taping application provides resilient support while limiting full stretch of the injured structure. Elastic tape also allows normal changes in structure girth while maintaining compression; thus vital circulation to the area involved is not jeopardized.

BONY PROMINENCES

These are superficial bony areas with little overlying soft tissue. These areas require special care when taping as the prominent points easily develop skin blisters and abrasions under tape because they lack significant subcutaneous protection.

If tape strips are applied too tightly over these areas, the compression can result in compromised circulation, neural compression or acute pain leading to impaired performance.

USEFUL MNEMONIC FOR ASSESSMENT

As discussed in Chapter Three, before beginning any taping procedure it is important to assess the injured region in order to determine the most appropriate treatment and taping application. The following material is presented in a format designed to facilitate a simple, quick assessment of the degree of injury in three areas: **sprains, strains** and **contusions** (bruising). Similar charts for specific injuries are included in Chapters Six to Nine following each of the taping techniques illustrated. Should there be any uncertainty concerning the severity of any particular condition, further medical evaluation and investigation must be sought. It is the responsibility of the taper to recommend such further medical care.

We have devised a simple order of assessment steps with a mnemonic to assist the reader. **T.E.S.T.S.** stands for:

T TERMINOLOGY: proper names, synonyms and other pertinent information for identifying an injury condition.

E ETIOLOGY: relative mechanisms, causative factors, prevalence.

S SYMPTOMS: subjective complaints of the injured patient including a description of the injury; objective physical findings which can be measured by the taper.

T TREATMENT: includes early and later phases of first aid, manual therapy, taping; medical follow-up when necessary.

S SEQUELAE: possible complications that can result if the original condition is left untreated, is poorly treated or if adequate medical follow-up is not pursued.

The following three charts are intended to clarify the classification and degree of injury. They outline the various aspects of treatment and put taping procedures in perspective relative to the total treatment plan. Taping alone is not a definitive treatment, but rather a protection and means to facilitate a safe, speedy recovery.

NOTE:

Using the mnemonic R.I.C.E.S., one can easily remember the basic treatment elements for acute soft tissue injuries: **R**est, **I**ce, **C**ompression, **E**levation, **S**upport.

	FIRST DEGREE	SECOND DEGREE	THIRD DEGREE
Terminology	FIRST DEGREE: fibre damage with little or no elongation	SECOND DEGREE: overstretch with partial tearing causing moderate to major elongation	THIRD DEGREE: complete rupture
Etiology	mild direct or indirect stress to a ligament	moderate stress to a ligament	severe stress to one or more ligaments
Symptoms	• some pain at rest possible • some pain on active movement (in direction of trauma) • some pain on resisted movement (in direction of trauma) • some pain on passive movement (in direction of trauma) • pain on stress testing of injured ligament • some swelling • some discolouration • no instability • minimal loss of function	• localized and/or diffuse pain even at rest • pain on active movement (direction of injury) • pain on resisted movement (multi-directional) • pain on passive stretch (in direction of injury) • exquisite tenderness at site of injury • significant swelling • discolouration not always present immediately • marked pain on stressing ligament • demonstrable laxity on stress testing • slight to significant loss of structural integrity • mild to moderate loss of dynamic function	• often less painful than 2nd degree due to rupture of ligament • marked swelling • discolouration common • significantly abnormal movement on stress testing • major loss of structural integrity • major loss of structural function
Treatment: early later	• R.I.C.E.S. first 48-72 hours • taped support • therapeutic modalities • range of motion continued therapy including: • taped support: 3–10 days until pain-free • activity permitted (with taping) if no pain • strengthening exercises (isometric at first) • proprioception	• R.I.C.E.S. for first 48-72 hours • taped support allowing for possible swelling • non-weightbearing first 48 hours. • therapeutic modalities continued therapy including: • mobilization if stiff • transverse friction massage if local swelling and stiffness • isometric strengthening • modified activity for 2–3 weeks followed by closely monitored return to activity if pain-free with taped support • continue taping 4–6 weeks • proprioceptive reeducation crucial to avoiding reinjury • total rehabilitation programme to restore range of motion, flexibility, strength, balance coordination and proprioception	• R.I.C.E.S. for first 48–72 hours • taped support • often requires surgery, bracing or casting with fibreglass or plaster physiotherapy including: • therapeutic modalities • mobilizations if stiff (postimmobilization) • flexibility • strengthening (isometric at first with the joint in neutral position) • modified exercise programme to maintain fitness level throughout treatment • gradual pain-free reintegration programme with taped support • continued taped support for at least 4 months • ligaments require up to 1 year to regain full tensile strength • total rehabilitation programme as for 2nd degree with emphasis on proprioception: 2–3 months
Sequelae	• chronic pain at site of injury • reinjury • weakness • stiffness	• chronically unstable or 'lax' joint • chronic pain • reinjury • reduced proprioception • weakness • arthritic changes	• adhesions • prolonged disability • instability if ligament heals in a lengthened position • high probability of reinjury if rehabilitation is incomplete • weakness • reduced proprioception and reaction ability • arthritic complications

R.I.C.E.S.: Rest, Ice, Compress, Elevate, Support

STRAINS: INJURY TO ANY PART OF A MUSCULO-TENDINOUS UNIT

Terminology	FIRST DEGREE: fibre damage with little or no elongation	SECOND DEGREE: partial tearing of fibres causing moderate to major elongation	THIRD DEGREE: complete rupture
Etiology	• mild to moderate stress against muscle contraction • mild to moderate overstretching • unaccustomed activity • lack of warm-up	• moderate to severe stress against muscle contraction • moderate to severe overstretching • unaccustomed resisted, repetitive activity	• severe stress against a muscle contraction • explosive muscle contraction causing spontaneous contraction of the antagonist muscle during vigorous physical activity ('hamstring' strains in sprinters; calf strains in tennis players) • severe overstretching • improper warm-up and/or pre-activity stretching • weakened tendons from repeated cortisone injections
Symptoms	• mild local or diffuse pain • some swelling • some discolouration possible • pain on active contraction • increased pain on resistance • increased pain on passive stretch • pain on local palpation • minimal loss of function	• moderate to major pain, localized and/or diffuse • moderate swelling • discolouration not apparent if intramuscular • moderate to major pain on active contraction • moderate to severe pain on resistance • moderate to major weakness • moderate to severe pain on passive stretch • spasm • pain localized on palpation • moderate to major loss of function	• often minimal pain due to complete rupture • marked swelling • discolouration varies with injury site • no significant pain on active contraction • zero strength on selective testing • 'bunching' of muscle can cause bump & hollow deformity • total loss of function
Treatment: early later	• R.I.C.E.S. for first 48-72 hours • taping to prevent full stretch and to give elastic support to musculo-tendinous unit (compression taping over muscle belly if injury site is in muscle bulk). See compression taping for calf Chapter 6 or quads Chapter 7 • weight-bearing only if pain-free • therapeutic modalities continued therapy including: • flexibility exercises • progressive strengthening • controlled activity with taped support • continue taping for 1-3 weeks • transverse friction massage for adhesions • rapid return to full pain-free activity • total rehabilitation programme for strength, flexibility and proprioception	• R.I.C.E.S. for first 48-72 hours • taping as for 1st degree; compression taping over muscle belly if injury site is in muscle belly • non-weightbearing during first 48 hours or until pain-free • therapeutic modalities • active contraction of antagonist (opposite) muscle to induce relaxation, flexibility and eliminate spasm continued therapy including: • flexibility exercises • strengthening exercises • transverse friction massage for adhesions • modified exercise programme to maintain fitness • gradual pain-free reintegration to full activity with taped support • continue taping for 3-6 weeks	• R.I.C.E.S. for first 48-72 hours • taping support to shorten structure: 3 weeks immobilization • surgery or casting in a shortened position often recommended therapy including: • therapeutic modalities • modified exercise programme to maintain fitness • flexibility exercises • strengthening exercises: begin with isometric progressing to eccentric and concentric • gradual reintegration to full pain-free physical activity with taped support; continue taping for 8-12 weeks • total rehabilitation programme for flexibility, strength and proprioception
Sequelae	• chronic pain • scarring • inflexibility • weakness • reinjury	• chronic pain • scarring • inflexibility • weakness and inhibition • prone to tendinitis • reinjury possibly causing complete rupture	• scarring • inflexibility • weakness • significant loss of function should healing take place while muscle is in a lengthened position • reduced reaction ability

R.I.C.E.S.: Rest, Ice, Compress, Elevate, Support

CONTUSIONS: CRUSHING INJURY TO SOFT TISSUE (CAN BE INTRAMUSCULAR OR INTERMUSCULAR)

Terminology	FIRST DEGREE: minor soft tissue crushing	SECOND DEGREE: moderately strong direct blow causing moderate trauma and bruising	THIRD DEGREE: major soft tissue damage
Etiology	mild direct or indirect blow causing bruising	moderately strong direct blow causing moderate trauma and bruising	hard direct blow – usually to the muscle belly, causing severe trauma and major bleeding
Symptoms	• localized pain • minimal swelling • some discolouration possible if intra-muscular • range of motion usually not significantly affected • some pain on active movement • some pain on resistance • some pain on passive stretch • tender on palpation • athletic ability generally not restricted	• significant diffuse and localized pain • noticeable swelling • discolouration if intermuscular • restricted range of motion due to pain and swellling • moderate to major pain on active contraction • major pain on resistance • weakness • major pain on passive stretch • tender on palpation • moderate loss of function	• severe pain • extensive swelling • discolouration if inter-muscular • very limited range of motion • pain on active contraction • marked spasm • often a palpable deformity at injury site or a palpable fluid mass if intra-muscular
Treatment: early later	• R.I.C.E.S. for first 48–72 hours • immediate taped support: See compression taping for calf Chapter 6 or quads Chapter 7 • active contraction of opposing muscles to restore full flexibility continued therapy including: • flexibility • strengthening • transverse friction massage for adhesions • controlled activity with compressive support • continue taping 3–10 days until pain-free	• R.I.C.E.S. for first 48–72 hours • immediate taped support: See compression taping for calf Chapter 6 or quads Chapter 7 • therapeutic modalities continued therapy including: • cautious progression of pain-free strengthening exercises • active contraction of antagonist muscles to induce pain-free stretching of the injured muscle	• R.I.C.E.S. for first 48–72 hours • immediate taped support. See compression taping for calf Chapter 6 or quads Chapter 7 • complete rest • leg injuries require crutches • therapeutic modalities • active isometric contraction of antagonist muscles peripheral to injury site to induce pain-free stretching continued therapy including: • flexibility exercises • no massage during first 3 weeks • transverse friction massages for adhesions only in later remodelling stage (4 weeks) • cautious progression of pain-free strengthening exercises with taped support • controlled, gradual pain-free progression of activity with taped support • continued compression for at least 4–8 weeks
Sequelae	• cramping • scarring • loss of flexibility • reinjury	• traumatic myositis ossificans (bone formation within the muscle) often caused by aggressive, premature massage, heat and/or stretching • scarring • inflexibility • permanent weakness • deformity	• traumatic myositis ossificans (bone formation within the muscle) often caused by aggressive, premature massage, heat, and/or stretching • scarring • inflexibility • permanent weakness • deformity • risk of spontaneous rupture

R.I.C.E.S.: Rest, Ice, Compress, Elevate, Support

REFERENCES

1. Watson T. Tissue healing. Electrotherapy on the web. Available online at: www.electrotherapy.org.

2. Lederman E. Assisting repair with manual therapy. In: The science and practice of manual therapy. Edinburgh: Elsevier, 2005: 13-30.

3. Hardy MA. The biology of scar tissue formation. Phys Ther 1989; 69: 1014-1024.

4. Rarick GL, Bigley GK, Ralph MR. The measurable support of the ankle joint by conventional methods of taping. J Bone Joint Surg 1962; 44A: 1183-1190.

5. Fumich RM, Ellison AE, Guerin GJ et al. The measured effects of taping on combined foot and ankle motion before and after exercise. Am J Sports Med 1981; 9: 165-170.

6. Bunch RP, Bednarski K, Holland D et al. Ankle joint support: a comparison of reusable lace on brace with tapping and wrapping. Physician Sports Med 1985; 13: 59-62.

7. Leanderson J, Ekstam S, Salomonsson C. Taping of the ankle – the effect on postural sway during perturbation, before and after a training session. Knee Surg Sports Traumatol Arthrosc 1996; 4: 53-56.

8. Taimela S, Kankaanpaa M, Luoto S. The effect of lumbar fatigue on the ability to sense a change in lumbar position. A controlled study. Spine 1999; 13: 1322-1327.

9. Ivins D. Acute ankle sprain: an update. Am Fam Physician 2006; 10: 1714-1720.

10. Popovic N, Gillet P. Ankle sprain. Management of recent lesions and prevention of secondary instability. Rev Med Liege 2005; 60: 783-788.

11. Carter AF, Muller R. A survey of injury knowledge and technical needs of junior Rugby Union coaches in Townsville (North Queensland). J Sci Med Sport 2008; 11: 167-173.

12. Palmer T, Toombs JD. Managing joint pain in primary care. J Am Board Fam Pract 2004; 17(suppl): S32-42.

13. Perryman JR, Hershman EB. The acute management of soft tissue injuries of the knee. Orthop Clin North Am 2002; 33: 575-585.

14. Bleakley CM, McDonough SM, MacAuley DC et al. Cryotherapy for acute ankle sprains: a randomized controlled study of two different icing protocols. Br J Sports Med 2006; 40: 700-705.

15. MacAuley D, Best T. Reducing risk of injury due to exercise. BMJ 2002; 31: 451-452.

16. Worell TW. Factors associated with hamstring injuries. An approach to treatment and preventative measures. Sports Med 1994; 17: 338-345.

17. Hubbard TJ, Denegar CR. Does cryotherapy improve outcomes with soft tissue injuries? J Athl Train 2004; 39: 278-279.

18. Petersen J, Holmich P. Evidence based prevention of hamstring injuries in sport. Br J Sports Med 2005; 39: 319-323.

19. MacAuley D. Do textbooks agree on their advice on ice? Clin J Sports Med 2001; 11: 67-72.

20. Bleakley C, McDonough S, Macauley D. The use of ice in the treatment of acute soft tissue injury: a systematic review of randomized controlled trials. Am J Sports Med 2004; 32: 251-261.

21. MacAuley DC. Ice therapy: how good is the evidence? Int J Sports Med 2001; 22: 379-384.

22. Watts BL, Armstrong B. A randomised controlled trial to determine the effectiveness of double tubigrip in grade 1 and 2 (mild to moderate) ankle sprains. Emerg Med J 2001; 18: 46-50.

23. Kerkhoffs GM, Struijs PA, Marti RK et al. Different functional treatment strategies for acute lateral ankle ligament injuries in adults. Cochrane Database Syst Rev 2002; 3:CD002938.

24. Bullock-Saxton JE, Janda V, Bullock MI. The influence of ankle sprain injury on muscle activation during hip extension. Int J Sports Med 1994; 15: 330-334.

Most taping applications are variations on basic key taping strategies. The differences in taping techniques lie in the manner and application of each strip of tape and the type of taping material used. Each particular taping strategy has to meet the requirements and needs of the patient, remain within the rules of the sport, if relevant, take into account the type of joint and related structures to be taped, as well as the type and severity of the injury.

When tape is to be applied circumferentially around a limb it is usually applied from distal (lower) to proximal (upper) so as not to adversely affect blood flow. The veins have valves in them which stop the blood from flowing in the reverse direction and these valves could be damaged if blood is forced back into them by taping from proximal to distal. When taping circumferentially from proximal to distal (as in closing up) the tape must be applied lightly.

This short chapter will familiarize the reader with the most common elements of our taping strategies, including the functional descriptive names of individual strips of tape, their purpose and method of application.

The strips illustrated include:
- anchors
- stirrups
- vertical strips
- 'butterfly' or check-reins
- locks
- figure of eight
- compression
- closing up.

TAPE TEARING/RIPPING

Before attempting these strips it is worthwhile learning how to tear tape efficiently. Tape tearing is an acquired skill and not as easy as it sounds or looks when done by an experienced taper! The types of tape that are readily torn are non-elastic tape (zinc oxide) and cohesive bandage. The steps shown in Figures 5.1 and 5.2 will be useful in learning this practical skill.

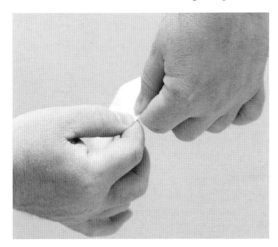

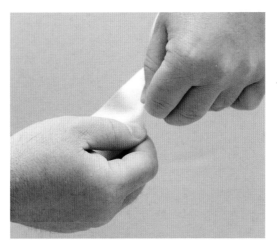

1 Pinch the tape edge firmly with your thumbnails (back to back and perpendicular to the tape)

2 Make a sudden jerking movement by sharply shearing your hands in opposite directions while maintaining tension on the tape edge.

PREPARATION OF PRACTICE STRIPS

To acquire taping skills, practice strips can be prepared. Because the precise applications of figure of eight and locking strips are tricky to learn, it is advisable to apply numerous practice strips to perfect the technique. Practice strips can be applied to the limb as though they were regular strips and the various complicated techniques can be practised without wasting tape. By experimenting with the 'take-off' angle and the degree of lateral shearing, the taper can learn to accommodate for the varieties of ankle shapes and thickness. It is important to be able to control the direction of the strip and thus adapt the final supporting result.

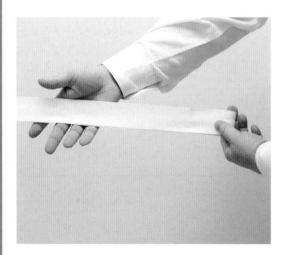 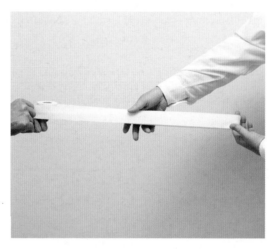 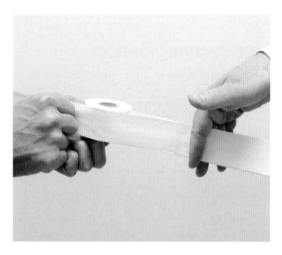

1   Unroll 1 metre (3 ft) of tape and have a helper hold it at one end.

2   Hold the tape with two fingers (slightly separated) with your left hand while your helper unrolls another 1 metre of tape.

3   Guide these two pieces of parallel tape (sticky side in) so that they meet without overlapping.

4   While maintaining tension on the tape, gently press one strip against the other throughout the length of the tape while controlling the tension to avoid wrinkles and overlapping.

5   Remove your fingers from the loop end of the tape and stick the sides together.

6   Finish sticking the other end of the tape and remove from the roll, leaving one side 15 cm (6 in) longer than the original piece with one sticky side.

COMMONLY USED TAPE STRIPS

ANCHORS

Description: The first tape strip applied to each tape job. They may be non-elastic or elastic, depending on the expansion requirements of underlying structures.

Purpose: To form a base for subsequent supporting strips of tape.

Method: Place these strips around the circumference of the limb to be supported, above and below the injury. They must be placed directly on the skin (after appropriate preparation) and they must follow the natural anatomical contours for optimal adherence.

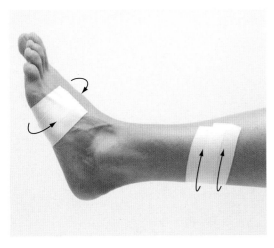

Open, non-elastic tape anchors.

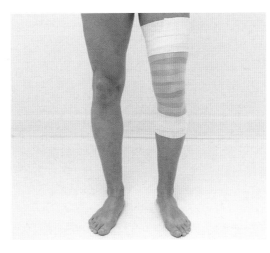

Elastic tape anchors.

STIRRUPS

Description: A U-shaped loop of non-elastic tape.

Purpose: To directly support an injured ligament and to support (in this case) the sub-talar joint.

Method: Attaching one end to the anchor, place the tape so that a lateral and medial component lends stability. Pull the tape tighter on the injured side and attach firmly to the anchor.

NOTE:
Tension must be maintained until the strip is firmly attached.

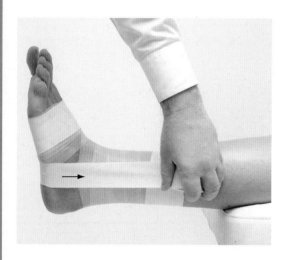

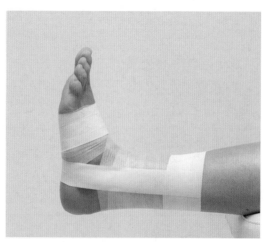

VERTICAL STRIPS

Description: Non-elastic tape strips applied under tension from one anchor to another.

Purpose: To limit mobility by drawing the distal segment of the injured structure towards the proximal.

Method: Affix one end of the vertical strip to the distal anchor. Apply tension to the tape over the injured structure and affix the tape strip to the proximal anchor. The structure should now be in a shortened position.

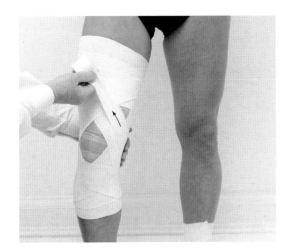
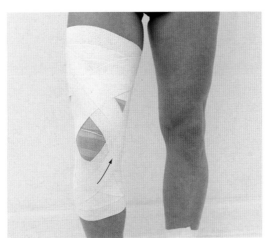

NOTE:
Proper position of the injured limb is crucial to effective application.

NOTE:
Maintain contact over the origin of the tape strip at the anchor while applying tension across the injury site so that the tape strip does not pull off.

'BUTTERFLY' OR CHECK-REIN

Description: A combination of three or more vertical strips applied at angles of between 10° and 45° to each other, placed at the axis of rotation of the joint to be taped. These strips can be of either non-elastic or elastic tape depending on the injured structure and the goal of the taping.

Purpose: To restrict movement in more than a simple uniplanar direction, as so often found in normal motion. This 'butterfly' or check-rein can resist stresses with inherent torsion components as well as those that are purely unidirectional.

Method: Steps in applying 'butterfly' strips:

NOTE:
The axis of the three strips lies directly over the joint line.

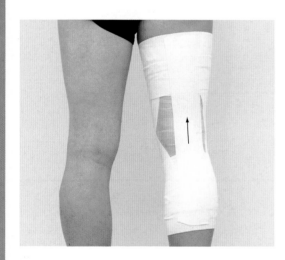

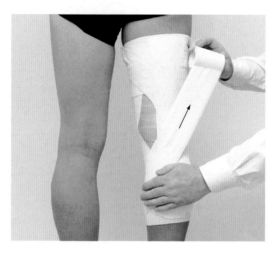

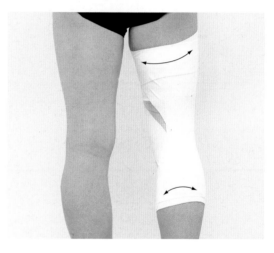

First strip: in a truly vertical position from the distal anchor to the proximal anchor.

Second strip: in a slightly rotated fashion in one direction.
Third strip: the same, but in the opposite direction to the second strip.

Final step: re-anchor these strips to hold the check-reins in place.

Key Taping Techniques

5

LOCKS

Description: A non-elastic tape strip attached firmly to the underlying tape reinforcing stabilization of the injured structure.

Purpose: To reinforce stability of the sub-talar joint and the talo-crural joint medially and laterally while allowing functional movements.

Method: Strong tension is applied at specific points in the application to reinforce the tape job, to ensure that selected ranges of motion are limited at end of range of motion to avoid overstressing of the injured structure.

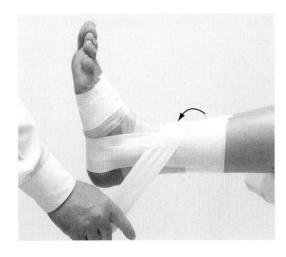
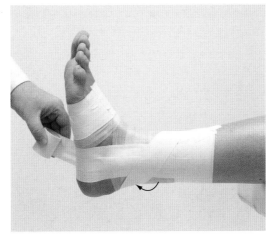
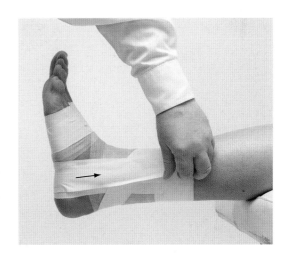

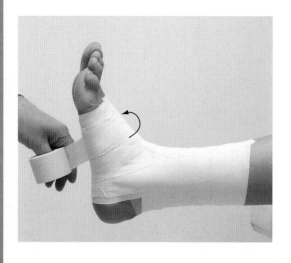

FIGURE OF EIGHT

Description: A strip of non-elastic tape forming a figure of eight; usually applied as one of the last strips in an ankle or thumb taping.

Purpose: To give added stability; to cover any remaining open areas and/or tape ends; to close the tape application neatly.

Method: Apply the tape by encircling one segment of the limb in one direction before crossing over to encircle the adjacent segment in the opposite direction, thus forming a figure of eight.

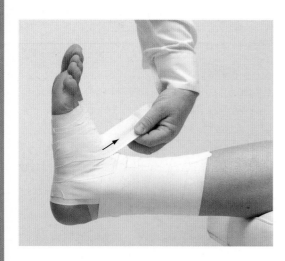

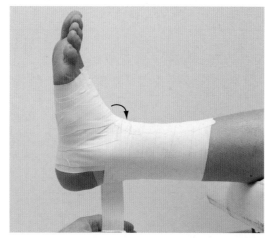

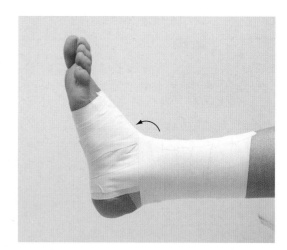

COMPRESSION STRIPS

Description: Elastic adhesive tape strips applied with localized compression over a muscle injury.

Purpose: To provide ample compression forces localized to the injured area without compromising circulation; limit swelling; decrease the chances of further damage to the injury site; allow continued activity.

Method:

1. Apply one layer of elastic adhesive tape directly to the skin of the injury site (Comfeel™ may be applied as a barrier), with minimal tension, from distal to proximal.

2. Apply pressure strips by pulling the tape in opposite directions until fully stretched, and then apply firmly directly over the injury site, covering about 50% of the limb circumference. Maintain the pressure on the limb and **gradually** release the tape to ensure tension over the injury site. Continue around the limb **without tension** (to avoid a tourniquet effect) until the ends overlap.

3. Repeat the compression strips, with each subsequent strip overlapping the previous one by half until the entire injured area (distal to proximal) is covered.

NOTE:
It is essential that the tension is released completely before closing each tape strip.

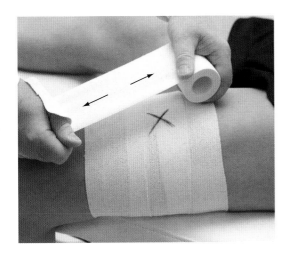
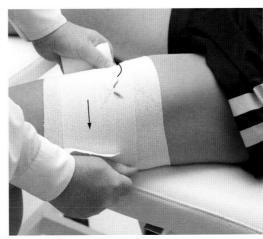

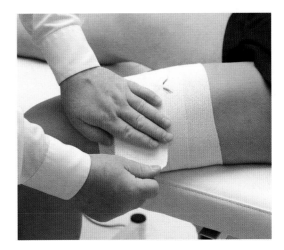

CLOSING-UP STRIPS

Description: Lightly placed strips of elastic or non-elastic tape, which cover any remaining open areas or tape ends, neatly finishing the taping job.

Purpose: To reduce the risk of skin blisters by covering all open areas. It also makes the tape job less likely to unravel during sporting activity.

Method: Lightly apply the strips of tape around the circumference of the limb, with one-third to one-half width of overlap.

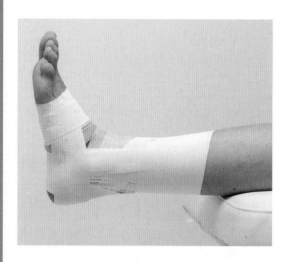
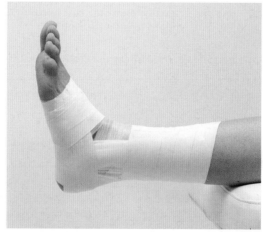
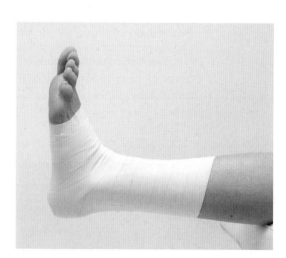

Section 2

PRACTICE

The procedures for taping the majority of sports injuries are illustrated in this and the following chapters. The purpose of these procedures is to provide protection while allowing functional movement, thus preventing further damage to the injured structure or adjacent areas. Inherent in each approach, and essential to accurate assessment of every injury, are medical diagnosis, treatment and appropriate follow-up.

T.E.S.T.S. charts in this section put each taping technique into perspective relative to total injury management. They include key points under the headings of **T**erminology, **E**tiology, **S**ymptoms, **T**reatment and **S**equelae. These charts are meant as helpful guides and are not to be considered as in-depth analyses with all possible complications.

A thorough understanding of the techniques illustrated in these chapters, combined with experience in handling a wide range of injuries, will enable the taper to adapt and apply effective taping techniques to the many unusual and/or challenging situations which inevitably arise.

In this and the following chapters, details on the following items will prove useful:

- specific purpose of each taping technique
- conditions appropriate for specific applications
- list of materials
- special notes
- positioning for taping procedure
- illustrated procedure
- highly informative sidebar tips
- a sample condition (injury) in a T.E.S.T.S. chart form

ANATOMICAL AREA: FOOT AND ANKLE

FOOT AND ANKLE TAPING TECHNIQUES

The articulations of the foot and ankle are numerous and complex. The joints of the foot and curvature of the arches of the foot permit adaptation to irregular terrain. These joints offer suppleness and shock absorption through elasticity. This varied bony architecture and mobility predisposes to different types of injuries. Taped support can alleviate many stresses related to these conditions.

The **talo-crural** (the true ankle) joint is mainly responsible for dorsiflexion and plantarflexion while the **sub-talar joint** allows more lateral mobility – inversion and eversion (sideways deviation) – permitting the foot to adapt to all angles of incline or slope. This relatively mobile **ankle joint complex** is dependent on numerous ligaments for its stability, and on tendons for its dynamic support. Forces through this relatively fragile joint make it vulnerable to stresses. The ankle is most easily injured during weight-bearing activities which require quick changes of direction.

A variety of taping techniques are highly effective in supporting both ligamentous and musculo-tendinous conditions related to the ankle joint. With the application of proper taping techniques, the athlete can rapidly resume normal competitive activity and/or intense training.

SURFACE ANATOMY

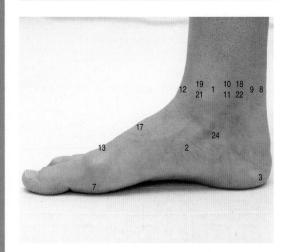

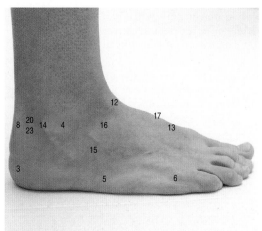

Right ankle and foot, from the lateral side. The most prominent surface features are the lateral malleolus, the tendo-calcaneus at the back and the tendon of tibialis anterior at the front.

Right ankle and foot, from the medial side. The most prominent surface features are the medial malleolus, the tendo-calcaneus at the back and the tendons of tibialis anterior and extensor hallucis longus at the front.

BONES

1. Medial malleolus
2. Tuberosity of navicular
3. Tuberosity of calcaneus
4. Lateral malleolus
5. Tuberosity of base of 5th metatarsal
6. Head of 5th metatarsal
7. Sesamoid bone

TENDONS

8. Tendo calcaneus (Achilles)
9. Flexor hallucis longus
10. Flexor digitorum longus
11. Tibialis posterior
12. Tibialis anterior
13. Extensor hallucis longus
14. Peroneus longus and brevis
15. Extensor digitorum brevis
16. Extensor digitorum longus

ARTERIES

17. Dorsalis pedis
18. Posterior tibial

VEINS

19. Great saphenous
20. Small saphenous

NERVES

21. Great saphenous
22. Posterior tibial
23. Sural

LIGAMENTS

24. Sustentaculum tali

Anatomical area: foot and ankle

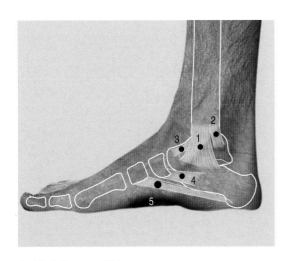

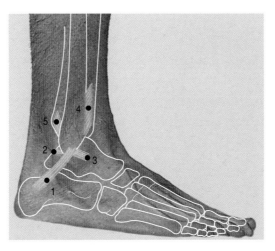

Ankle joint: lateral aspect.
1 Calcaneo-fibular ligament,
2 posterior talo-fibular ligament,
3 anterior talo-fibular ligament,
4 anterior tibio-fibular ligament,
5 posterior tibio-fibular ligament.

Ankle joint: medial aspect.
1 Medial ligament,
2 posterior tibio-talar ligament,
3 anterior ligament,
4 plantar calcaneo-navicular ligament,
5 long plantar ligament.

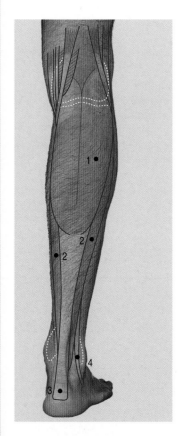

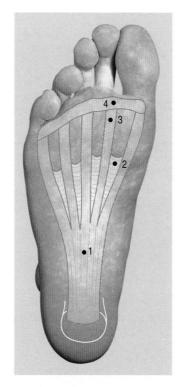

Posterior aspect of lower leg and heel: Superficial muscles
1 Gastrocnemius
2 Soleus
3 Tendo calcaneus
4 Peroneus longus

Sole of foot: Plantar fascia
1 Plantar aponeurosis
2 Transverse bands
3 Digital bands
4 Superficial transverse metatarsal ligament

TAPING FOR TOE SPRAIN

Purpose

- Support of first metatarsophalangeal (MTP) joint
- Allows moderate flexion and some extension
- Limits the range of flexion, extension and adduction

Indications for use

- Sprains of the first metatarsophalangeal (MTP) joint.
- For medial collateral ligament sprain: abduct the toe and reinforce the medial restraining tape strips.
- For plantar ligament sprain (hyperextension injury): reinforce the **X** on the plantar surface to limit extension.
- For lateral collateral ligament sprain: reinforce with buddy taping to the first toe (for an example of buddy taping with fingers, see p. 209).
- For dorsal capsular sprain (hyperflexion): reinforce the **X** on the dorsal surface to limit flexion.
- Hyperflexion of first MTP joint: 'turf toe'.
- Contusion of the first MTP joint: 'jammed toe', 'stubbed toe'.
- Painful bunions.
- Hallux rigidus.

NOTES:

- The styloid process at the base of the fifth metatarsal is a sensitive area vulnerable to pressure, pain and blisters if tape is too tight.
- To avoid constriction, minimal tension must be used when wrapping circumference anchors.
- Application of lubricant to adjacent toes and/or the inside of the toe box of the shoe will prevent chafing.
- Trimming toenails will lessen the risk of irritation.
- Careful application of a minimum amount of tape is particularly important when taping for sports that require tight-fitting shoes or boots.

For additional details regarding an injury example, see T.E.S.T.S. chart (p. 61).

MATERIALS

Razor
Skin toughener spray/adhesive spray
2 cm (³⁄₄ in) non-elastic tape

Positioning

Sitting on treatment table with injured foot slightly overhanging the end of the table.

Procedure

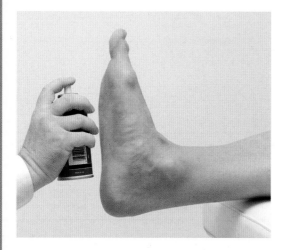
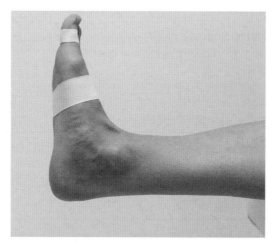

1 Make sure the area to be taped is clean and relatively hair free; shave if necessary

2 Check skin for cuts, blisters or areas of irritation before spraying with skin toughener or spray adhesive.

3 Place an anchor of 2 cm non-elastic tape around the distal toe at the base of the toenail.

4 Place two anchors of 3.8 cm (1½ in) non-elastic tape around the instep and arch of the foot.

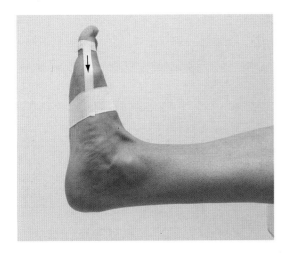

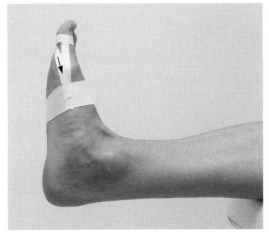

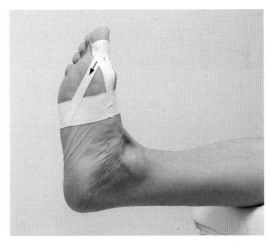

5 Place a longitudinal supporting strip of 2 cm non-elastic tape from distal to proximal between the anchors.

NOTE:
Abduct the toe slightly and apply two strips with tension when taping for a medial collateral ligament sprain or bunions.

6 Begin a plantar **X** with a longitudinal strip diagonally from the **lateral** aspect of distal anchor to the medial aspect of the proximal anchor on the plantar aspect of the first MTP joint.

7 Cross this with a second strip from the medial aspect of the distal anchor, crossing the MTP joint at its midpoint on the plantar aspect.

NOTE:
Extension must be adequately limited with this X when taping hyperextension injuries.

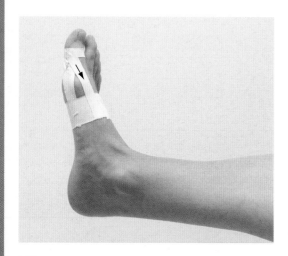

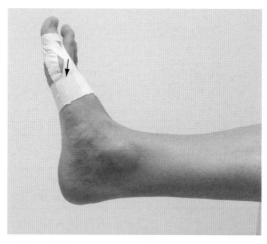

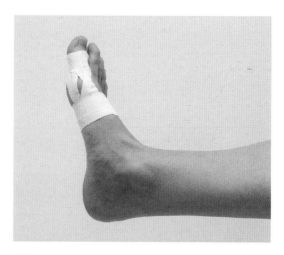

8 Begin dorsal **X** with a 2 cm strip from the medial aspect of the distal anchor to the dorsal aspect of the proximal anchor.

9 Finish the dorsal **X** by crossing this strip from the lateral aspect of the distal anchor to the medial aspect of the proximal anchor, crossing the **X** over the dorsal MTP joint.

NOTE:

Flexion must be adequately limited with this X when taping for hyperflexion injuries.

10 Close up taping with light circumferential strips covering sites of the original anchors with 2 cm tape, starting proximally and moving distally, overlapping each previous strip by half.

11 Test tape for adequate restriction to ensure functional pain-free support.

NOTE:

The colour, temperature and sensation must be checked to verify that circulation has not been compromised.

ANATOMICAL AREA: FOOT AND ANKLE

INJURY: TOE SPRAIN

T ERMINOLOGY
- sprain of medial or lateral collateral ligament
- hyperflexion with capsular injury
- hyperextension with capsular injury
- sprain of the plantar ligament
- 'jammed' toe; 'stubbed' toe; 'turf' toe

E TIOLOGY
- sudden forced flexion, extension or abduction
- sudden longitudinal impact against a hard surface
- repetitive dorsiflexion of great toe (as in kicking a ball or sprinting) can cause a synovitis
- chronic sprain
- inadequately supportive footwear on artificial turf

S YMPTOMS
- tenderness of the first metatarsophalangeal joint
- often swollen
- active movement testing:
  a. pain on end-range flexion with hyperflexion injuries
  b. pain on end-range extension with hyperextension injuries
  c. pain on end-range abduction with medial collateral ligament sprain
- passive movement testing:
  a. pain on end-range flexion with hyperflexion injuries
  b. pain on end-range extension with hyperextension injuries
  c. pain on end-range abduction with medial collateral ligament sprain
- resistance testing (neutral position): no significant pain on moderate resistance

- stress testing:
  a. pain with or without laxity on medial (or lateral) stress with 1st- and 2nd-degree sprains of the medial (or lateral) collateral ligaments
  b. instability with less pain in 3rd-degree sprains

T REATMENT
Early
- R.I.C.E.S.
- taping for: **Toe Sprain** (see p. 57)
- therapeutic modalities

Later
- continued treatment including:
  - therapeutic modalities
  - passive mobilizations if painful or stiff
  - flexibility
  - strengthening exercises
  - gradual pain-free reintegration to sports activities with taped support
  - a shoe with stiff soles for reinforcement may be necessary
  - dynamic weight-bearing activity should start only after 45° of pain-free dorsiflexion is attained

S EQUELAE
- pain
- chronic swelling
- diminished mobility
- weakness
- chronic synovitis
- flexor hallucis longus tendinitis
- degenerate changes leading to hallux rigidus (stiff first toe)

R.I.C.E.S. : Rest, Ice, Compress, Elevate, Support

6

Foot and Ankle

ANATOMICAL AREA: FOOT AND ANKLE

TAPING FOR LONGITUDINAL ARCH SPRAIN/PLANTAR FASCIITIS

Purpose

- supports plantar aspect of foot (functionally shortens and reinforces the longitudinal arches – medial more than lateral)
- permits plantarflexion mobility
- limits extension (dorsiflexion) of the midtarsal joints

Indications for use

- plantar fasciitis
- acute or chronic midfoot sprains
- flat feet or fallen arches
- medial knee pain caused by flat feet
- bone spurs
- shin splints

MATERIALS

Razor
Skin toughener spray/adhesive spray
2.5 cm (1 in) non-elastic tape
3.8 cm (1½ in) non-elastic tape

NOTES:

- Remember the foot will spread when weight bearing, rendering the tape job tighter.
- Pressure on the base of the fifth metatarsal can cause pain.
- Pressure on the neighbouring blood vessels can cause pain and compromise circulation.
- Tape thickness must be kept to a minimum for sports requiring tight-fitting footwear.
- Excessive medial tension must be avoided, especially in ankles predisposed to inversion sprain.

For additional details regarding an injury example, see T.E.S.T.S. chart (p. 67).

Positioning

Either lying prone with knee slightly bent or sitting facing the taper (as illustrated).

Procedure

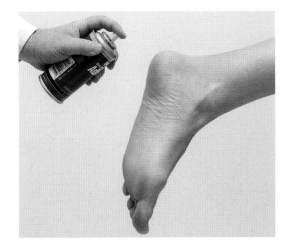

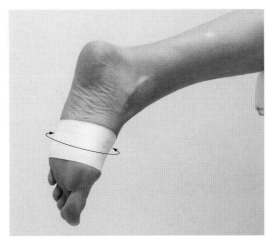

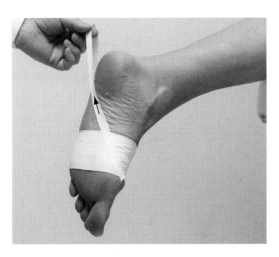

1 Make sure the area to be taped is clean and relatively hair free; shave if necessary.

2 Check skin for cuts, blisters or areas of irritation before spraying with skin toughener or spray adhesive.

3 Place anchor strips of 3.8 cm non-elastic tape using very light tension around the foot at the level of the heads of the metatarsals to allow for splaying of the metatarsals when weight bearing.

4a Using firm tension, place a strip of 2.5 cm non-elastic tape from the head of the first metatarsal under the arch of the foot and around the heel.

Longitudinal arch sprain/plantar fasciitis

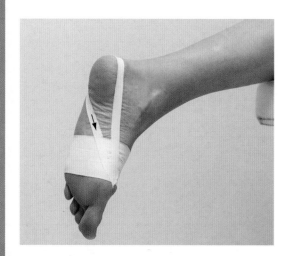

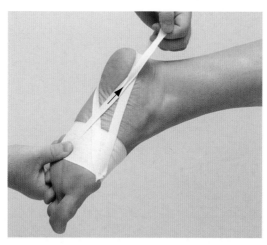

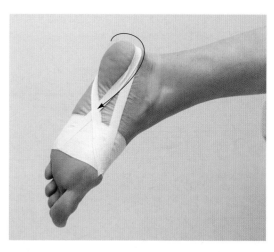

4b Finish at the medial aspect of the first metatarsal, tensioning the tape to shorten the medial arch.

5a Starting from the lateral aspect of the anchors plantar surface, apply a second strip with strong tension, crossing the transverse arch diagonally around the heel.

5b Pass behind the heel without tension and finish over the lateral aspect of the head of the fifth metatarsal.

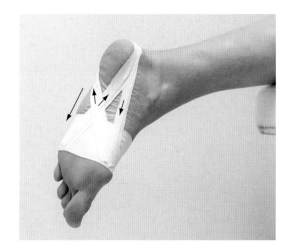

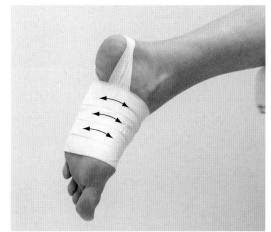

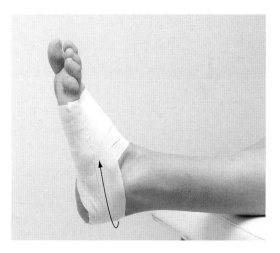

 6 Repeat steps 4a,b and 5a,b as necessary.

7 Close up with circumferential strips of 3.8 cm non-elastic tape. Apply with a light pressure as the natural spread of the foot on weight bearing will tighten the tape job. Start at the head of the metatarsals, overlapping each previous tape by at least a half, progressing towards the heel.

8 Test for degree of support. There should be a significant reduction of pain on weight bearing.

 NOTE:
If ankle stability is a concern a figure of eight can be added; see steps 9 and 10.

9 Apply two overlapping horizontal strips of 3.8 cm non-elastic tape.

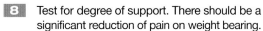 **NOTE:**
Apply lubricant and heel and lace pads to the anterior ankle and posterior heel if friction spots are likely to develop.

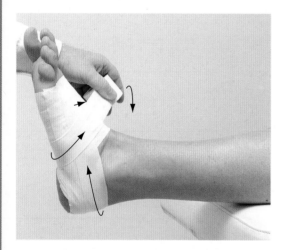

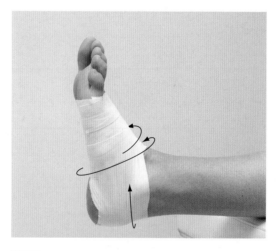

10a Start figure of eight strip on the dorsum of the foot (top) from lateral to medial. Pass under the arch and pull up on the lateral side of the foot to resist inversion.

10b Continue around behind the heel and complete the figure of eight.

ANATOMICAL AREA: FOOT AND ANKLE

CONDITION: PLANTAR FASCIITIS

T ERMINOLOGY
- chronic or acute inflammation of plantar fascia
- heel spurs

E TIOLOGY
- intrinsically tight plantar fascia
- poor foot biomechanics
- sudden change in training routine, i.e. distance, frequency, speed, change of terrain
- poorly supportive or new footwear
- secondary to midfoot sprain or tarsal hypomobility

S YMPTOMS
- pain and tenderness on plantar aspect of foot, more concentrated on the medial aspect of the calcaneal attachment
- active movement testing: no significant pain on weight bearing
- passive movement testing: pain on full stretch of fascia
- resistance testing (neutral position): no significant pain
- pain on first steps after resting
- pain on weight bearing, particularly on push-off

T REATMENT
- therapy including:
- R.I.C.E.S.
- therapeutic modalities
- Support: taping: **Longitudinal Arch** (see p. 62).
- Rest: reduction of weight-bearing activities
- selective stretching of tendo Achilles and plantar fascia
- strengthening of plantar muscles
- heel lifts can be helpful in acute phase (a bevelled doughnut depression will reduce pressure pain)

S EQUELAE
- injury often becomes chronic without correct treatment
- development of heel spurs
- tight tendo Achilles complex
- may predispose to shin splints
- orthotics may be indicated

R.I.C.E.S. : Rest, Ice, Compress, Elevate, Support

6

Foot and Ankle

ANATOMICAL AREA: FOOT AND ANKLE

TAPING FOR: PREVENTIVE PROPHYLACTIC ANKLE SPRAINS

Purpose

- offers bilateral ankle stability with specific reinforcement of the lateral ligaments
- restricts inversion and some eversion
- allows almost full range of dorsiflexion and plantarflexion

Indications for use

- preventive taping to protect lax ligaments and 'weak' ankles
- final stages of ankle sprain rehabilitation, when less specific ligamentous reinforcement is sufficient
- chronic inversion sprains
- for chronic medial sprains (deltoid ligament): reverse strips (steps 6–8, 10–12, 14 and 16) to reinforce medial rather than lateral support

NOTES:

- It is essential to confirm the site of any injury or laxity prior to taping, so that appropriate reinforcements can be made.
- The athlete should be asked if they have any taping preferences. e.g. light tape or tight. Tension can be adjusted to suit during the procedure.
- Pressure on the base of the fifth metatarsal can cause pain. Pressure on the neighbouring blood vessels can cause pain and compromise circulation.
- Proprioception retraining is extremely important to ensure a total recovery programme.

MATERIALS

Razor
Skin toughener spray/adhesive spray
Lubricant
Heel and lace pads
Underwrap/Comfeel™
3.8 cm (1½ in) or 5 cm (2 in) non-elastic tape ±
5 cm elasticized tape for closing

For additional details regarding an injury example, see T.E.S.T.S. chart (p. 61).

Positioning

Lying supine (face up) or long sitting (knees extended) with ankle held at 90° angle over the end of the table and supported at the midcalf (a 90° angle is the 'normal standing' angle).

 TIP:
The taping surface should be high enough that the taper can work comfortably without risking back strain.

Procedure

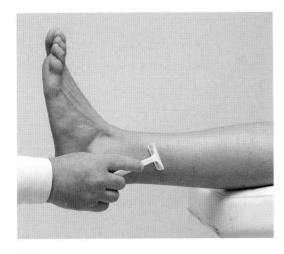

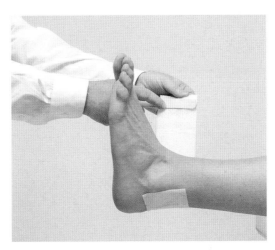

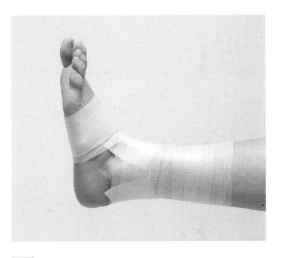

 Make sure the area to be taped is clean and relatively hair free; shave if necessary.

Check skin for cuts, blisters or areas of irritation before spraying with skin toughener or spray adhesive.

3 Apply lubricant to lace and heel pads to the two *'danger'* areas where blisters frequently occur.

 TIP:
Cover the Achilles tendon including its attachment to the heel and superficial extensors.

4 Apply underwrap to the area to be taped.

NOTE:
Comfeel™ may be applied prior to lace and heel pads and would negate the need for underwrap. The more contact between the tape and the skin, the more likely you are to have an unyielding tape job.

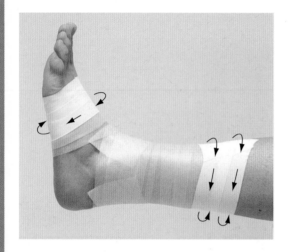

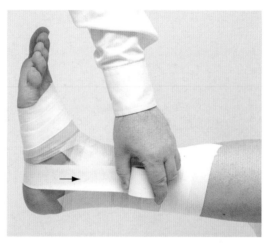

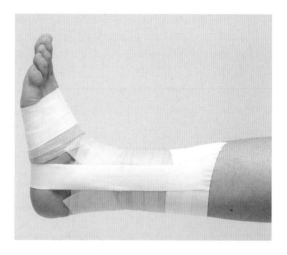

 5 Using light tension, apply two overlapping, circumferential anchor strips of 3.8 cm non-elastic tape at the forefoot and two below the calf bulk (at the musculo-tendinous junction).

 6 Apply a stirrup of 3.8 cm non-elastic tape. Starting from the upper anchor medially, pass under the calcaneum and pull up slightly on the lateral side to end on the upper anchor laterally.

 TIP:
Make sure the ankle is held at an angle of 90° throughout this procedure and make sure you secure the stirrup to the anchor before tearing the tape from the roll.

 TIP:
When applying the anchor strips midcalf, be sure that the strip is held horizontally at the back and wraps around the natural contours, rising up to cross more superiorly on the anterior surface.

 NOTE:
These anchors must be in direct contact with the skin to ensure support.

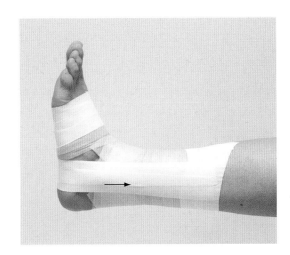

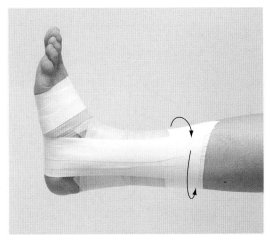

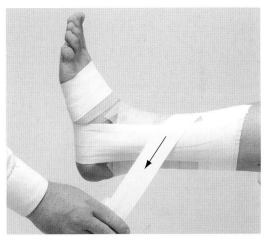

7 Apply a second and third stirrup (if necessary) slightly anterior to the preceding one.

8 Repeat the proximal anchor (5) to hold the end of the stirrups in place.

9a Apply the first heel/ankle lock beginning on the anterior shin, pass towards the lateral aspect of the ankle superior to the malleolus.

Foot and Ankle

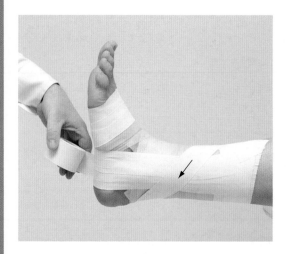

9b Continue cautiously behind the Achilles tendon and under the heel.

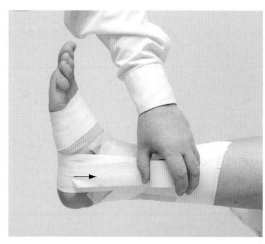

9c Pull up over the lateral side, applying strong tension, and fix securely on the lateral upper anchor. Alternatively this can be pulled over the area of the anterior talo-fibular ligament region and back toward the origin.

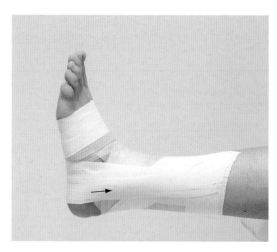

10 Repeat the lock.

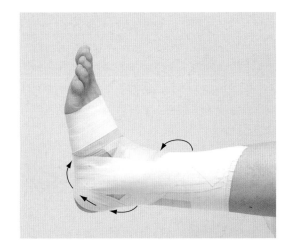

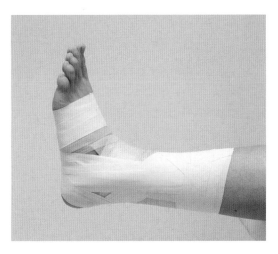

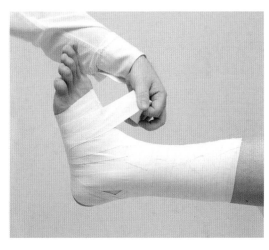

11 Apply medial lock by reversing this strip and finishing on the medial side for added stability.

12 Begin closing up the tape job from the top (lightly), ensuring all gaps (windows) are covered in order to avoid blisters.

13a Apply a simple figure of eight to close and support the taping. Start anteriorly, crossing medially without tension.

TIP:
Apply medial tension only when pulling up on the medial side.

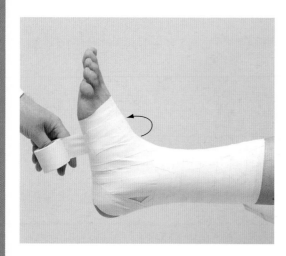

13b Pull the tape down towards the medial aspect of the arch.

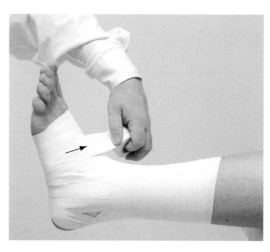

13c Pass under the foot and pull up with firm tension over the lateral side before crossing the ankle.

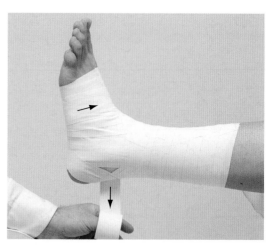

13d Bring the tape horizontally behind the Achilles tendon, finishing anteriorly, crossing the starting point.

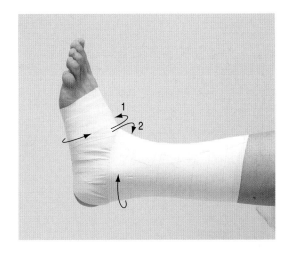

14 Complete the closing up strips, covering the forefoot if not already completely enclosed.

NOTE:
A second figure of eight can be applied to offer greater support or to cover any remaining open areas.

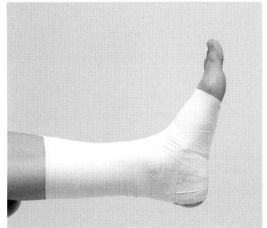

15 **a.** Test the degree of restriction. **b.** Inversion should be significantly restricted.
c. Plantarflexion should be limited by at least 30°.

NOTE:
Medial view of the finished tape job is shown in this photograph.

ANATOMICAL AREA: FOOT AND ANKLE

TAPING FOR: ANKLE SPRAIN/CONTUSION: ACUTE STAGE

Purpose

- gives lateral stability through splinting and compression
- permits some plantarflexion and dorsiflexion
- controls swelling without compromising arterial and nerve supply (removal of the safety strip permits easy release of tension in case of progressive swelling)

Indications for use

- acute (inversion) lateral ankle sprain
- acute (eversion) medial ankle sprains: reverse strips to support medially damaged structures
- acute postcast removal
- splinting for suspected ankle fracture: use less tension and apply equally to both sides
- acute ankle contusion: apply tension to injured side

NOTES:

- Ensure that the correct diagnosis has been made. **If in doubt, refer!**
- Take care to apply adequate, localized compression over the basic taping without compromising circulation. (Take care not to cause a tourniquet effect.)
- Ensure that the athlete has been thoroughly instructed in (and understands) the immediate care for the first 72 hours: R.I.C.E.S.
- Check regularly for signs of numbness, swelling or cyanosis (blueish colouring) of the toes.
- Should the tape become too tight due to continued swelling (even after R.I.C.E.S.) loosen the tape or completely reapply.

MATERIALS

Razor
Skin toughener spray/adhesive spray
3.8 cm (1½ in) non-elastic tape
Foam/felt/gel pad cut into a U or J shape
5 cm (2 in) or 7.5 cm (3 in) elastic adhesive bandage

For additional details regarding an injury example, see T.E.S.T.S. chart (p. 36–38).

Ankle sprain/contusion: acute stage

Positioning

Lying supine (face up) with a cushioned support under the midcalf and with the injured ankle held at 90° throughout this procedure (a 90° angle is the 'normal standing' angle).

Procedure

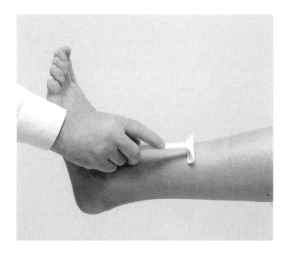

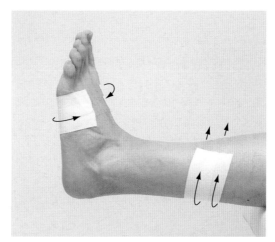

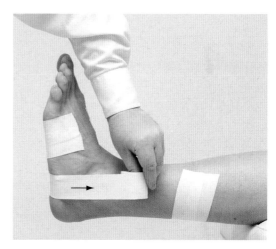

1 Make sure the area to be taped is clean and relatively hair free; shave if necessary

2 Check skin for cuts, blisters or areas of irritation before spraying with skin toughener or spray adhesive.

3 Apply two open anchors of 3.8 cm non-elastic tape around the lower third of the calf. Be sure to leave an opening at the front.

TIP:
Ensure the anchors at horizontal at the back of the calf apply to the skin then follow the natural contours of the skin.

4 Apply two anchors around the midfoot, leaving an open space on the dorsum (top).

5 Apply a stirrup of 3.8 cm non-elastic tape from the upper anchor on the medial side, cover the posterior edge of the medial malleolus, pass beneath the heel and slightly behind the lateral malleolus. Pull up strongly to apply specific tension over the lateral side and affix the tape to the upper anchor laterally.

NOTE:
When taping medially injured structures, this stirrup is applied in reverse, starting on the lateral side and pulling up strongly on the medial side.

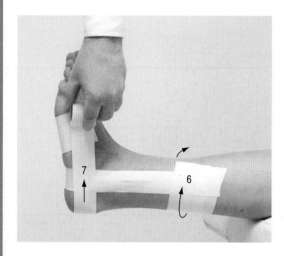

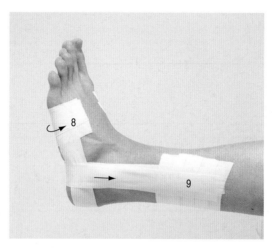

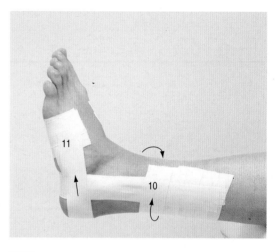

6 Apply an open anchor around the upper end of this stirrup, overlapping the original anchor by a half anteriorly.

7 Apply a horizontal strip from the anchor on the medial side of the foot, passing around the calcaneum below the level of the malleoli, applying tension as it is applied to the lateral side of the anchor.

8 Stabilize this horizontal strip with a vertical forefoot anchor, overlapping the previous anchor by a half.

9 Apply a second stirrup as in step 5, overlapping the previous stirrup by half anteriorly.

10 Anchor the stirrup as in step 6, moving lower on the calf and covering the previous anchor by a half.

11 Apply a horizontal strip overlapping the previous strip by half proximally, pulling strongly on the lateral side.

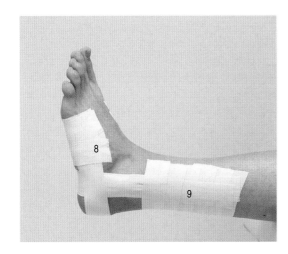

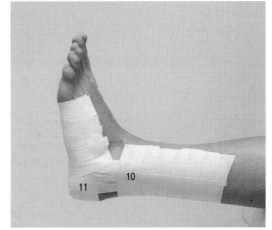

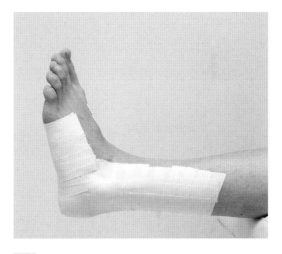

12 Repeat steps 8 and 9, overlapping the previous strips and always pulling strongly on the lateral side.

13 Repeat steps 10 and 11, overlapping again in the same manner.

14 Repeat steps 8–11 until all the gaps are covered.

TIP:
Be sure the ankle is kept at an angle of 90° throughout this procedure.

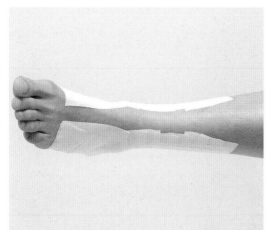

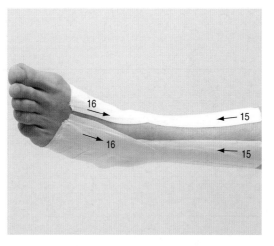

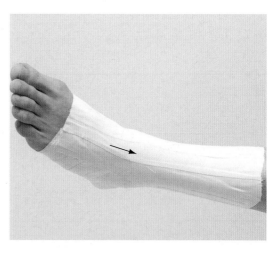

NOTE:
None of the strips should overlap anteriorly.

 15 Apply a pair of vertical strips, lightly covering the tape ends on either side of the gap anteriorly from the shin to the ankle.

16 Apply a second pair of parallel strips from the forefoot, pulling up slightly and covering the previous strips at the ankle.

17 Gently test the degree of restriction. There must be no laxity on lateral stressing. The pain should be significantly reduced on testing.

18 Apply a final, **single**, safety strip to close the remaining area.

TIP:
Allow slight plantarflexion while applying this strip to ensure continuous adhesion of the tape at the front of the ankle.

NOTE:
This safety strip is easily loosened in case of progressive swelling.

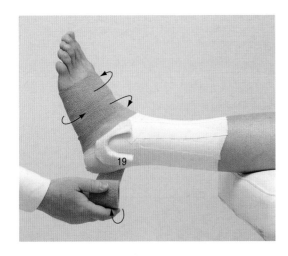

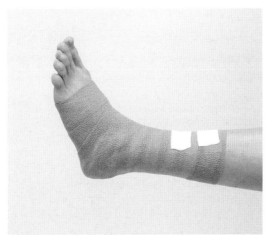

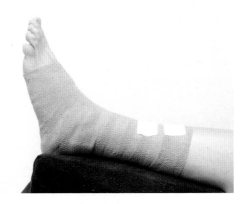

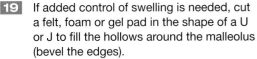 If added control of swelling is needed, cut a felt, foam or gel pad in the shape of a U or J to fill the hollows around the malleolus (bevel the edges).

20a Apply an elasticized bandage to hold it in place using a figure of eight pattern.

20b Stretch the elastic wrap each time as it crosses the lateral side and relax the tension while covering the medial side. Continue with gradually diminishing tension until the bandage covers the entire tape job.

21 Keep the foot elevated as much as possible during the first 48–72 hours.

TIP:
Cushions, pillows or rolled-up towels can be placed under the mattress if an appropriate bolster is not available.

 NOTE: THIS TAPE JOB IS NOT DESIGNED FOR WEIGHT-BEARING ACTIVITIES!

6

Foot and Ankle

ANATOMICAL AREA: FOOT AND ANKLE

TAPING FOR LATERAL ANKLE SPRAIN: REHABILITATION STAGE

Purpose

- offers lateral stability with specific reinforcement
- prevents inversion
- restricts end-range plantarflexion and some eversion
- allows almost full dorsiflexion and functional plantarflexion

Indications for use

- lateral ankle sprains (INVERSION sprain)
- injuries of the calcaneo-fibular and the anterior talo-fibular ligaments: in combination, the most common ankle sprain
- for medial ankle sprains (deltoid ligament): use a horseshoe instead of a J shape on the medial side in step 6 and reverse steps 9–11 and 15–16 for medial instead of lateral reinforcement

NOTES:

- Ensure that the injury has been properly evaluated by a competent sports medicine specialist, and that X-rays have been taken, particularly if an avulsion fracture is suspected.
- DO NOT USE THIS TECHNIQUE FOR AN ACUTE ANKLE INJURY. It should only be applied when acute swelling has subsided (for acute ankle injury taping see appropriate guide).
- Placement of a felt horseshoe controls residual perimalleolar swelling, particularly useful in the subacute phase when localized swelling can become chronic.
- Partial weight bearing with crutches is recommended when starting to bear weight.
- Progression to full weight bearing is permitted only if pain free.
- Use of a heel lift assists 'push-off' and reduces the need for dorsiflexion range, allowing weight bearing with less effort and stress.
- Weight-bearing activities may be continued and progressed only if there is no pain **during** or **after** activity.

For additional details regarding an injury example see T.E.S.T.S. chart (p. 92).

MATERIALS

Razor
Skin toughener spray/adhesive spray
Underwrap/Comfeel™
Heel and lace pads
3.8 cm (1.5 in) non-elastic tape
2 cm (¾ in) felt, foam or gel pad cut into a U or J shape
2 cm (¾ in) heel lift
7.5 cm (3 in) elastic wrap

Taping is adapted throughout the progressive rehabilitation healing stages:

1. **subacute stage:** (48–72 hours post injury): support with felt J and heel lift while beginning to bear weight

2. **functional stage:** specific ligamentous support with reinforcement of stability for moderate to dynamic activity

3. **return to sport stage:** reintegration with support adapted to specific sports requirements ranging from training to competition.

Positioning

Lying supine (face up) or long sitting (with knees extended), support at midcalf with the foot off the end of the table. The ankle must be held at an angle of 90 ° throughout the taping technique (a 90° angle is the 'normal standing' angle).

Procedure

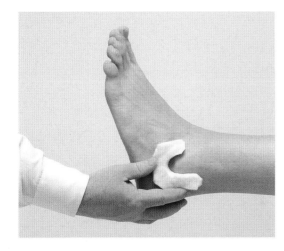

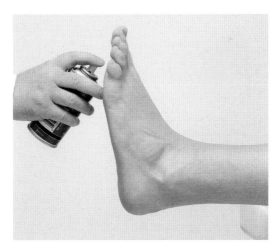

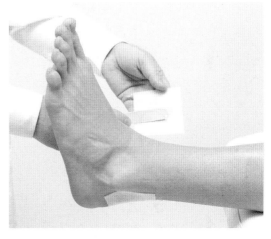

1 Make sure the area to be taped is clean and relatively hair free; shave if necessary.

2 To control swelling, cut a U or J shape to fill the hollows around the malleolus. Bevel the edges of the padding to form fit all contours.

3 Check skin for cuts, grazes, blisters or irritated areas prior to spraying with skin toughener or adhesive spray.

4 If repetitive activity is to be undertaken, apply lubricated heel and lace pads to the two 'danger' areas where blisters or tape cuts frequently occur.

TIP:
Keep the felt shape within reach ready to apply.

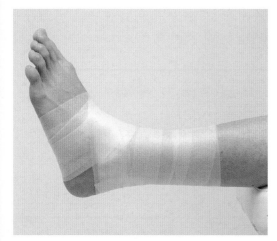

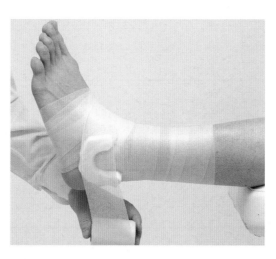

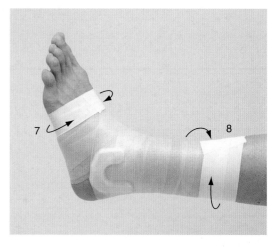

5 Apply underwrap or Comfeel™ to the area to be taped.

 TIP:
Allow for some splaying of the metatarsals to avoid discomfort when subjected to weight bearing.

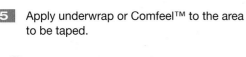 **NOTE:**
These anchors must be in direct contact with the skin to ensure support.

6 Attach the felt piece with an added figure of eight of underwrap.

7 Using light tension, apply two overlapping, circumferential anchor strips of 3.8 cm non-elastic tape below the calf bulk at the musculo-tendinous junction.

8 Apply two overlapping anchors around the forefoot.

 TIP:
Ensure the anchors are horizontal at the back of the calf, apply to the skin and then follow the natural contours of the skin.

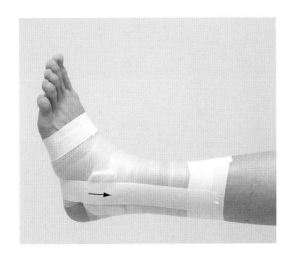

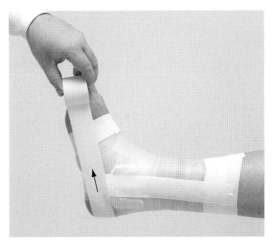

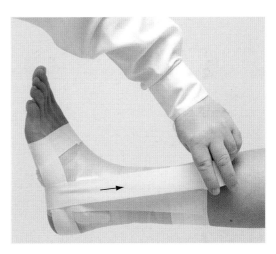

9 Apply a stirrup of 3.8 cm non-elastic tape from the upper anchor on the medial side, cover the posterior edge of the medial malleolus, pass beneath the heel and slightly behind the lateral malleolus. Pull up strongly to apply specific tension over the lateral side and affix the tape to the upper anchor laterally.

10 Starting on the medial side of the distal anchor, apply a horizontal strip passing behind the heel and covering the tip of the lateral malleolus. Put extra tension on the lateral side before re-attaching the tape to the distal anchor on its lateral side.

11 Apply a second stirrup as in step 9, overlapping the previous stirrup by half anteriorly.

TIP:
Ensure that the end of the tape is securely fixed to the anchor. Apply strong tension on the lateral side.

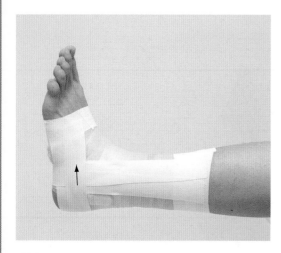

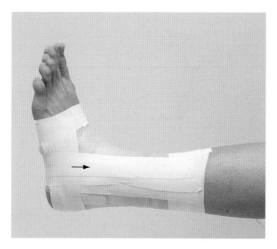

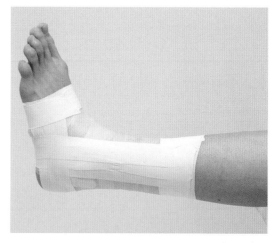

12 Apply a second horizontal strip as in step 10, overlapping the previous strip by half superiorly, covering the malleoli.

13 Apply a third stirrup as in step 9, overlapping the previous stirrup by half anteriorly.

14 Repeat the proximal and distal anchors.

TIP:

Always apply specific tension on the injured side.

NOTE:

These stirrups may be 'fanned' when the athlete is at the returning to sport stage of rehabilitation (see fanned stirrups, p. 94).

NOTE:

A third horizontal strip may be necessary when taping larger feet and when additional stability is required.

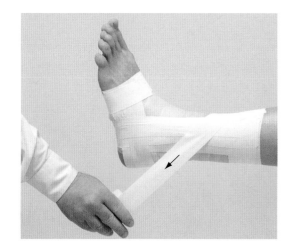

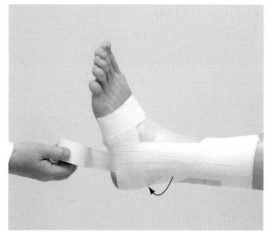

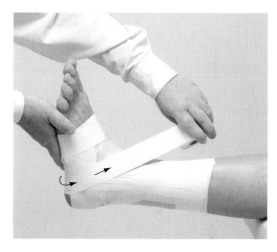

15a Apply the first lock: begin on the anterior shin, passing towards the lateral aspect of the ankle.

15b Continue behind the Achilles tendon and under the heel.

15c Then apply strong tension up over the lateral side to the lateral upper anchor.

NOTE:
Be careful to start with the appropriate angle so that the tape will follow the natural contours and end up in the appropriate place.

TIP:
Support and hold the foot in eversion (turned outwards) to ensure a shortened position for the ligaments while applying this important supporting strip.

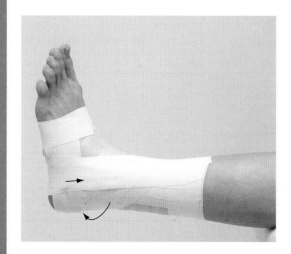

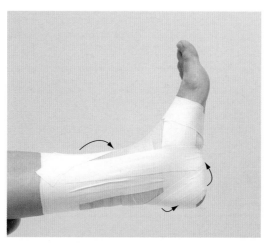

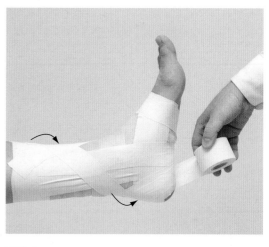

16 Repeat step 15 again on the lateral side, overlapping the previous strip by three-quarters.

17 View from lateral side.

17a To balance stability, apply the ankle lock on the medial side.

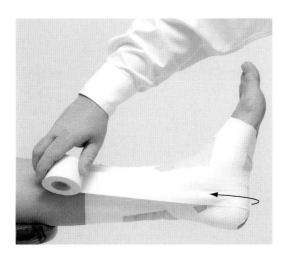

17b Less tension when pulling up on the medial side.

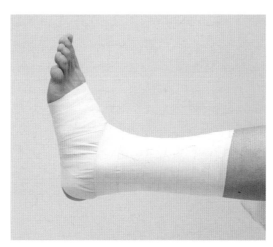

18 Re-anchor proximally.

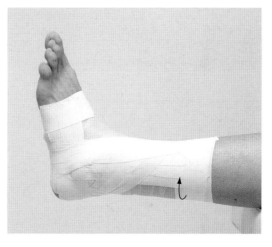

19 Close up the tape job by starting proximally and working distally, applying the strips lightly and overlapping each previous strip by half, ensuring all the gaps are covered in order to avoid blisters.

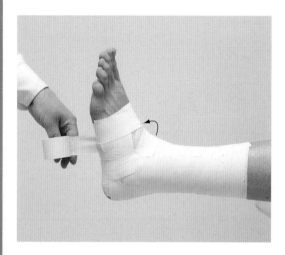

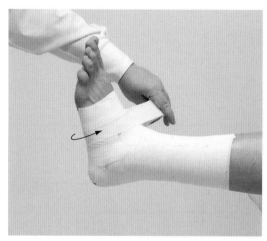

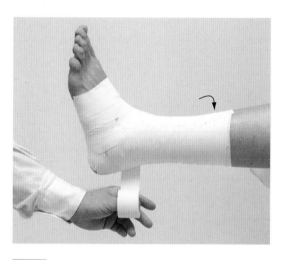

20a Apply a simple figure of eight to close and to reinforce the ankle tape. Use either non-elastic tape or an elastic adhesive bandage. Start anteriorly, crossing the ankle towards the medial aspect of the midfoot and pass under the foot.

20b Pull up with firm tension over the lateral side before crossing the ankle anteriorly with less tension.

20c Bring the tape horizontally behind the Achilles tendon.

TIP:

When pulling the EAB up with tension, hold the tape against the underlying tape below the point at which you want to apply the tension. Apply tension and then press up against the underlying tape. Move your point of contact to where you want to release the tension and hold the tape against the underlying tape here. Allow the EAB to recoil before proceeding with the technique.

NOTE:

If using an elastic adhesive bandage (EAB), allow the tape to recoil before applying, when no tension is needed.

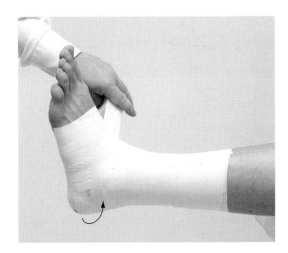

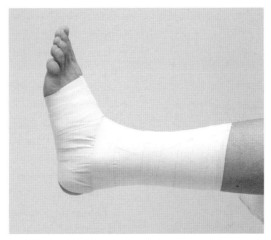

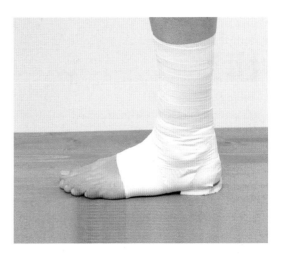

21 Finish anteriorly, crossing the starting point of the strip.

TIP:
Apply a second figure of eight if necessary to cover any open areas (overlap the first figure of eight by half).

NOTE:
For return to dynamic activity, a heel locking figure of eight or a reverse figure of eight can be applied in place of the regular figure of eight.

22 Complete the closing-up strips, covering the forefoot and distal anchors.

23 Starting gently, test the degree of inversion and plantarflexion restricted by the tape. Add reinforcement strips if these movements are not adequately limited or if they cause pain.

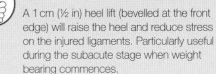

TIP:
A 1 cm (½ in) heel lift (bevelled at the front edge) will raise the heel and reduce stress on the injured ligaments. Particularly useful during the subacute stage when weight bearing commences.

NOTE:
Weight bearing and gradually increasing activity must only be permitted if pain free, both during and after activity.

ANATOMICAL AREA: FOOT AND ANKLE

INJURY: LATERAL ANKLE SPRAIN

(typically a combination of two ligaments: calcaneo-fibular and anterior talo-fibular)

T ERMINOLOGY
- see sprains chart (p. 36)
- inversion sprain
- 'turned' ankle

E TIOLOGY
- forced inversion with plantarflexion
- 'rolling over' on ankle
- often secondary to inadequate rehabilitation of a previous ankle sprain (reduced proprioception)
- the most commonly injured combination of ankle ligaments

S YMPTOMS
- local pain, swelling, discolouration and tenderness anteriorly and inferior to the lateral malleolus
- active movement testing: pain on plantarflexion with inversion
- passive movement testing: pain on plantarflexion with inversion
- resistance testing (neutral position): no significant pattern of pain with moderate resistance
- stress testing:
  a. pain, with or without laxity, on anterior 'drawer' test (forward gliding of the talus under the tibio-fibular mortice) indicates a 1st- or 2nd-degree sprain of the anterior talo-fibular ligament
  b. instability on forward displacement of the talus away from the lateral malleolus indicates a 3rd-degree sprain of the same ligament
  c. pain with or without some laxity on talar tilt test indicates a 1st- or 2nd-degree sprain of the fibulo-calcaneum
  d. instability or 'opening up' on the talar tilt test (often with little or no pain) is indicative of a 3rd-degree sprain of this ligament

T REATMENT
Early
- R.I.C.E.S.
- taping: first 48 hours: **Acute Ankle Injury (open basketweave)** (p. 76)
- therapeutic modalities
Later
- continued therapy including:
  a. therapeutic modalities
  b. transverse friction massage
  c. modified fitness activities
- progressive pain-free rehabilitation including:
  a. range of motion
  b. flexibility
  c. strength: non-weight bearing to weight bearing (endurance, then power)
  d. proprioception
- gradual painfree reintegration to sports activity with specific taping
- prevention of recurrent sprains

S EQUELAE
- anterior talo-crural and sub-talar instability if ligaments are not supported in a shortened position during healing phase
- weakness and/or tendinitis of peroneal muscles
- extensor digitorum longus is often injured simultaneously, predisposing to chronic residual weakness
- reduced proprioception
- repeated injury caused by poor proprioception and joint instability
- chronic swelling in the sinus tarsi and around the tip of the lateral malleolus

R.I.C.E.S.: Rest, Ice, Compress, Elevate, Support

ANKLE SPRAIN REHABILITATION – ADVANCED

SPECIAL ADAPTATIONS: SPORT-SPECIFIC ANKLE TAPING VARIATIONS

During the subacute and rehabilitation stage of ankle sprains, the tape job is adapted to the varying needs of the injury. Each tape job must be adjusted for the anatomy of the specific ligament, the degree of injury and the current stage of healing. As the athlete gradually returns to sports activity, his or her sport-specific requirements must also be accommodated.

NOTE:

Prior to initial application of ankle rehabilitation taping strategies, the ankle must be fully evaluated by a qualified person, for example a doctor, in order to identify the injured structures and to ensure that no other complications exist.

The following specialized strip adaptations may be used by the experienced taper in combination with the previously described strips to adapt to a wide range of situations.

Specialized strips for sports-specific techniques include:

- **fanned stirrups:** allows freer plantarflexion (useful when tight boots are required for a specific sports activity)
- **V-lock:** for extra heel stability (useful when the number of tape strips must be kept to a minimum, i.e. when the athlete must wear tight boots)
- **heel-locking figure of eight:** reinforces stability when the level of recovery permits a return to activity
- **reverse figure of eight:** reinforces stability without restricting plantarflexion (useful when plantarflexion is needed for sports participation)

SPECIALIZED STRIP: FANNED STIRRUPS

Purpose
- offers lateral support over three angles

Advantages
- allows more plantarflexion than straight basketweave stirrups
- mimics multi-angled ligamentous support
- allows minimal tape thickness over bony prominences
- useful when tight-fitting footwear is required as in figure skating, ice hockey, speed skating and downhill skiing where tape thickness over the malleoli must be kept to a minimum

Disadvantages
- reduced limitation of plantarflexion
- thickness is localized under heel

Procedure

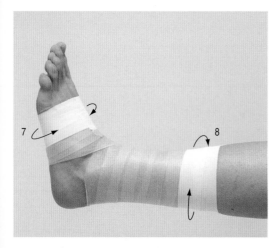

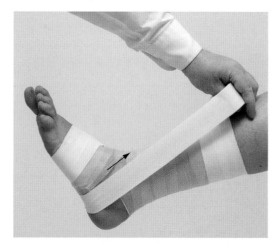

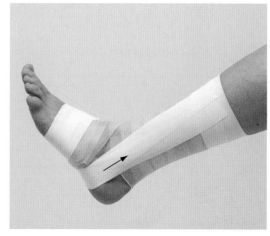

1 Begin taping by applying steps 1–8 (step 6 is optional) of **Ankle rehabilitation taping.**

2 Apply the first stirrup, starting from the upper anchor posteriorly on the medial side, passing under the heel, and pulling up with a strong tension on the finish more anteriorly on the lateral side of the anchor.

3 Attach the second stirrup, passing directly over the medial malleolus, passing under the heel and pulling up again with strong tension over the lateral malleolus to the anchor, ending slightly posterior than the first stirrup.

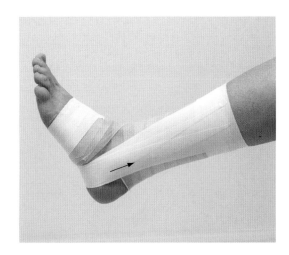

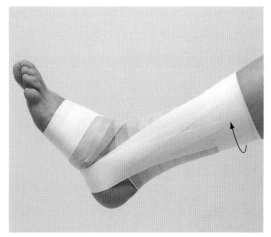

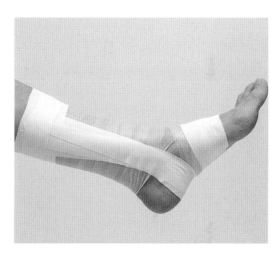

4 Apply the third stirrup, starting more anteriorly on the medial side and finishing posterior to the lateral malleolus on the lateral side.

5 Re-anchor these stirrups proximally (at the top) and proceed to the complete tape job as in steps 15–22 of **Ankle rehabilitation taping**.

View from the side.

TIP:
Ensure that the tape is high enough at the back so that it is at the same level when it crosses itself again anteriorly.

NOTE:
These stirrups are applied in combination with the horizontal strips to form a modified basketweave, offering more stable support, particularly for anterior and posterior (talo-fibular or deltoid) ligament sprains.

SPECIALIZED STRIP: V-LOCK

Purpose

- reinforces lateral stability
- locks the heel

Advantages

- offers a combination of lateral stability and heel locking with one single strip
- useful when tight-fitting footwear is required, as in figure skating, ice hockey, speed skating and downhill skiing where tape thickness over the malleoli (ankle bones) must be kept to a minimum

Disadvantages

- does not restrict talar tilt as effectively as the single ankle lock

Procedure

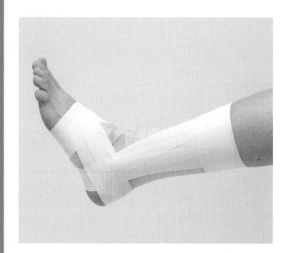

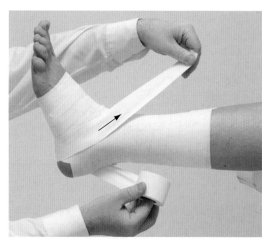

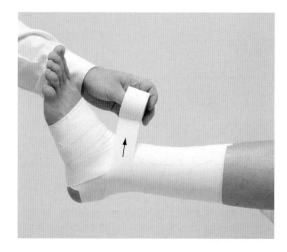

1 Begin taping by applying steps 1–8 (step 6 is optional) of **Ankle rehabilitation taping.** Fanned stirrups may also be used.

2 Place the tape under the heel before pulling up on the anterior end and affixing it to the upper anchor, anteromedially.

TIP:
Ensure that the foot is everted (pulled outward) by the pull of this step.

3 Gently wrap the roll of tape behind the heel, crossing low enough on the lateral side to cross over the lateral malleolus.

4 Pull the tape snugly across the lateral malleolus to the dorsum of the foot.

TIP:
Lateral shearing of the tape and careful attention to the 'take-off' direction will help in achieving the best taping 'line' without wrinkling the tape.

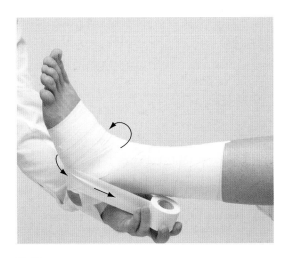

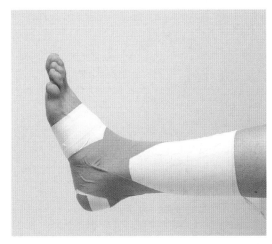

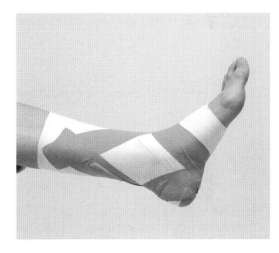

5 Wrap the tape without tension anteriorly across the ankle.

6 Pass medially to the plantar surface under the arch, going in a posterior direction.

7 Pull up strongly posterior over the lateral malleolus.

8 Attach the strip to the anchor posteromedially.

View from lateral side.

 TIP:
Repeated applications using practice tape strip will improve technique.

View from medial side.

 NOTE:
This strip can also be applied to the medial side for added stability and heel locking effect. Care must be taken not to allow inversion and to adjust the tension during application when taping for lateral ankle sprains.

SPECIALIZED STRIP: HEEL-LOCKING FIGURE OF EIGHT

Purpose

- offers added reinforcement with specific heel stabilization
- restricts full plantarflexion
- limits lateral mobility
- allows almost full dorsiflexion

Advantages

- useful in sports requiring more dorsiflexion and where there is less demand for extreme plantarflexion

Disadvantages

- restricts plantarflexion

Procedure

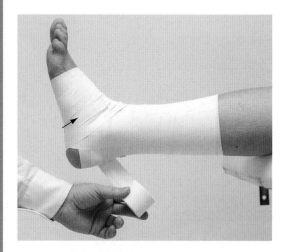

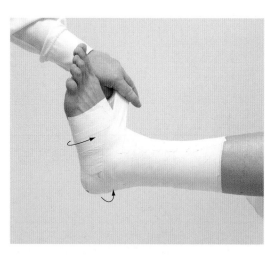

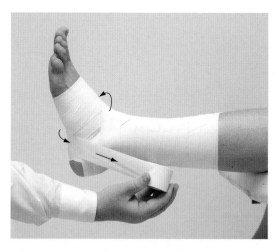

1 Begin taping by applying steps 1–5, 7–14 of **Ankle rehabilitation taping.** Fanned stirrups may also be used if desired.

2 Start strip on the dorsum of the foot, from lateral to medial, pass under the instep.

3 Pull up **strongly** on the lateral side.

4 Carefully cross the tape over the extensor tendons (without wrinkling) and pass horizontally behind the medial side to wrap around the Achilles tendon.

5 Cross the ankle anteriorly, moving down the medial side and under the instep, slightly posterior to the starting point. Angle the tape in a posterior direction under the plantar surface.

6 Pull the tape up and back with strong tension posterior to the lateral malleolus and pass behind the Achilles tendon.

TIP:
The ankle must be adequately dorsiflexed in order to allow the tape to pass posteriorly without bending, wrinkling or causing a pressure ridge.

TIP:
Ensure that strong tension is used when pulling up on the lateral side for all three strips.

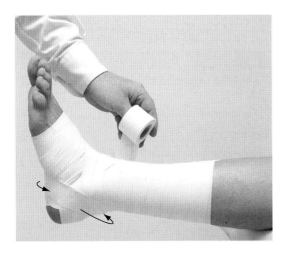

7 Continue carefully around the front of the ankle.

TIP:
Repeated application using a practice strip will aid in judging taping angles and will improve proficiency significantly.

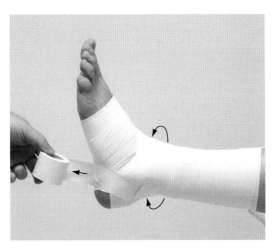

8 Return posteriorly behind the Achilles tendon again, this time crossing the heel from the medial side, using less tension, and pass under the instep.

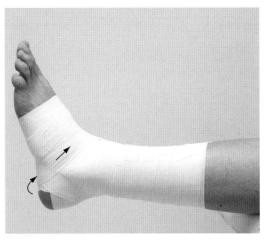

9 Pull up strongly on the lateral side to end by crossing the previous strips anteriorly.

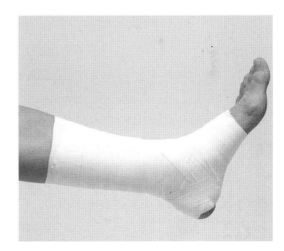

View from the medial side.

SPECIALIZED STRIP: REVERSE FIGURE OF EIGHT

Purpose

- offers added reinforcement with specific heel stabilization to a taped ankle
- restricts dorsiflexion
- limits lateral mobility of ankle and controls heel
- allows almost full plantarflexion

Advantages

- as this strip allows plantarflexion, it is particularly useful in sports that require a greater functional range of plantarflexion (basketball, volleyball, gymnastics, various track and field sports)
- controls heel from both sides

Disadvantages

- less stability in plantarflexion than offered by the other figure of eight strips

Procedure

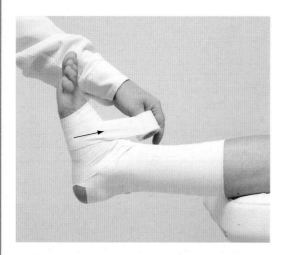

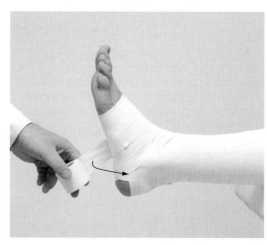

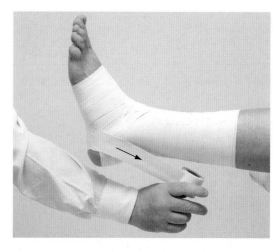

1. Begin taping by applying steps 1–5, 7–14 of **Ankle rehabilitation taping.** Fanned stirrups may also be used if desired.

2. Start strip on the dorsum of the foot, crossing from lateral to medial.

3. Pass tape under the instep heading in a posterior direction.

4. Pull the tape up and back with strong tension, moving behind the lateral malleolus (locking the heel laterally), and wrap the tape carefully around the Achilles tendon.

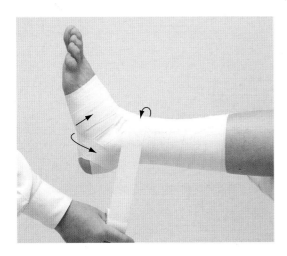

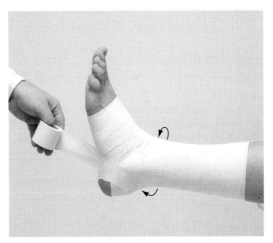

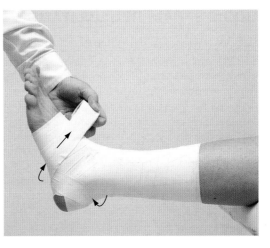

5 Bring the tape forward on the medial side. Carefully pass over the extensor tendons anteriorly and return posteriorly.

NOTE:
Be sure to avoid wrinkling or sharp angling of the tape when crossing these tendons.

6 Cross the Achilles tendon again, bringing the tape down across the medial side of the heel (locking it), then moving anteriorly under the plantar surface.

NOTE:
To severely limit dorsiflexion, position the ankle in slightly more plantarflexion and pull tightly when locking the heel from each side.

7 Pull up strongly on the lateral side and finish the strip by crossing over the starting point on the dorsum of the foot.

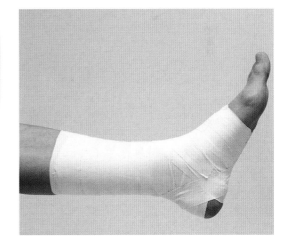

View from the medial side.

ANKLE SPRAIN REHABILITATION – ADVANCED

SUBSECTION FOR INDIVIDUAL LIGAMENT SPRAINS

The following is a detailed subsection on ankle sprains that may not be of interest to all readers. It is included to provide healthcare professionals intensively treating athletes with methods of specific taped support for isolated ligament sprains.

The **T.E.S.T.S.** charts in this section describe location and make-up of the individual ligaments in Terminology. The sequence and frequency of occurrence are included with Etiology, Symptoms, Treatment and Sequelae. This section illustrates how the rehabilitation taping elements are adjusted and adapted for the progressive stages of healing, the anatomy of the individual ligaments, and the varying demands of different sports.

The purpose of this subsection is to show how taping can be designed to support specific ligaments and how it can be constantly progressed and adapted to meet the changing needs of the healing structure and the varying demands of different sports.

Should any given technique not provide the necessary pain-free support, consider the following:

- question the original diagnosis and reassess the injury
- question the stage of healing: has the ankle suffered from further injury or an aggravation of the original injury, thereby prolonging the subacute stage?
- question the appropriateness of this taping technique for this injured structure and this stage of healing
- question your technique of application: could your skills be improved? (practise with a test strip)
- are the fundamental needs of the athlete met with adequate support yet sufficient mobility?

NOTE:
These procedures are intended as guidelines and suggestions and are by no means 'carved in stone'. They represent practical adaptations that have proven useful through theorization, application of knowledge and experience.

TIP:
To develop your skills and techniques, never stop questioning and adapting, as you apply anatomical and physiological principles to your taping.

Anterior talo-fibular ligament sprain

SPECIFIC ANKLE REHABILITATION TAPING FOR ISOLATED TALO-FIBULAR LIGAMENT SPRAIN

Positioning: seated, with the calf supported and the foot held at a 90 degree angle **BASIC STRIPS**	PROGRESSIVE STRIP ADAPTATIONS		
	SUB-ACUTE: (beginning to weightbear) • activity depends on stage of healing • how much swelling? • weightbearing only if no pain!	FUNCTIONAL: (moderate to dynamic activity) • adequate support for individual ligaments • enough mobility for moderate activity	RETURN TO SPORT: (training, then competition) • reinforced support • adaptations for specific needs of sport
BASIC PREPARATION (clean, shave, spray) underwrap anchors	• if swelling is likely, use a **felt 'J'**-lateral side (bevel the edges)	• if swelling persists, continue with **felt 'J'** • for increasing activity use **heel and lace pads**	• **use heel and lace pads**
LATERAL SUPPORT Stirrups	**modified basketweave** composed of: • **3 stirrups (vertical)** (start medially and pull up strongly on lateral side) • Interlock stirrups with **2 horizontal strips** (strong lateral pull)	• continue with **modified basketweave** (extra pull on lateral side for both horizontal and vertical strips)	• continue with **modified basketweave** (extra pull particularly on lateral horizontal strips) • for more mobility, **fanned stirrups** can be used
REINFORCEMENT Ankle locks	• **lateral locks** with main tension pulling up on last component (posterior vertical strip) • **medial V-lock** with main tension pulling from behind heel horizontally across medial malleolus	• continue with **1 lateral V-lock** **1 medial V-lock**	• continue with **1 lateral V-lock** **1 medial V-lock**
STABILIZATION Figure 8 variations	• **simple figure 8** (start medially and pull up strongly on lateral side) (ensure plantar flexion is restricted with this strip)	• **heel locking figure 8** for added stability (always pull up strongly on lateral side)	• continue with **heel locking figure 8** or • if more plantar flexion needed for sport, use **reverse figure 8** (ensure that end-range plantar flexion is limited with previous locking strips) • if tight, rigid boots are necessary, omit this step
CLOSING UP:	• add **felt heel-lift** for weightbearing	• **heel-lift** (optional)	**Purpose:** • *supports* anterior talo-fibular ligament • *prevents* inversion • *limits* inward rotation of foot, end-range eversion and end-range plantar flexion • *permits* functional plantar flexion

TIP:
Visualize location and direction of ligament being supported during tape application.

ANATOMICAL AREA: FOOT AND ANKLE

INJURY: ANTERIOR TALO-FIBULAR LIGAMENT SPRAIN

T ERMINOLOGY
- anterior portion of lateral ligamentous complex
- short, superficial band of fibres
- from the anterior portion of lateral malleolus forward to the neck of the talus
- see **anatomy illustration**, p. 55

E TIOLOGY
- forced inversion with plantarflexion
- 'rolling over' on ankle
- the most commonly injured ankle ligament
- often secondary to inadequate rehabilitation of a previous ankle sprain (reduced proprioception)
- often injured in combination with the fibulo-calcaneal ligament

S YMPTOMS
- local pain, swelling and discolouration
- tenderness just anterior to the lateral malleollus
- active movement testing: pain on plantarflexion with inversion
- passive movement testing: pain on plantarflexion with inversion
- resistance testing (neutral position): no significant pattern of pain with moderate resistance
- stress testing:
  a. pain, with or without laxity, on 'anterior drawer' test (forward gliding of the talus under the tibio-fibular mortice) indicates a 1st- or 2nd-degree sprain
  b. instability on forward displacement of the talus away from the lateral malleolus with or without pain can be indicative of a 3rd-degree sprain. An audible 'click' may be present

T REATMENT
Early
- R.I.C.E.S.
- taping, first 48 hours: **Acute ankle injury (open basketweave)** (p. 76)
- therapeutic modalities

Later
- continued therapy including:
  a. therapeutic modalities
  b. transverse friction massage
- modified fitness activities
- progressive pain-free rehabilitation including:
  a. range of motion
  b. flexibility
  c. strength: non-weight bearing to weight bearing (endurance, then power)
  d. proprioception
- gradual pain-free reintegration to sports activity with specific taping. **Ankle rehabilitation taping for isolated anterior talo-fibular ligament sprain: see p. 103 (when injured in combination with fibulo-calcaneal ligament, refer to lateral ankle sprain, p. 82)**
- prevention of recurrent sprains

S EQUELAE
- anterior talo-crural instability if ligament is not supported in a shortened position during healing phase
- weakness and/or tendinitis of peroneal muscles
- chronic residual weakness of extensor digitorum longus (often injured simultaneously)
- reduced proprioception
- repeated injury caused by poor proprioception and joint instability
- chronic swelling in the sinus tarsi

R.I.C.E.S. : Rest, Ice, Compress, Elevate, Support

SPECIFIC ANKLE REHABILITATION TAPING FOR ISOLATED CALCANEO-FIBULAR LIGAMENT SPRAIN

Positioning: seated, with the calf supported and the foot held at a 90 degree angle **BASIC STRIPS**	PROGRESSIVE STRIP ADAPTATIONS		
	SUB-ACUTE: (beginning to weightbear) • activity depends on stage of healing • how much swelling? • weightbearing only if no pain!	FUNCTIONAL: (moderate to dynamic activity) • adequate support for individual ligament • enough mobility for moderate activity	RETURN TO SPORT: (training, then competition) • reinforced support • adaptations for specific needs of sport
BASIC PREPARATION (clean, shave, spray) underwrap anchors	• if swelling is likely, use a **felt 'J'**-lateral side (bevel the edges)	• if swelling persists, continue with **felt 'J'** • for increasing activity use **heel and lace pads**	• use heel and lace pads
LATERAL SUPPORT Stirrups	**modified basketweave** composed of: • **3 stirrups (vertical)** (start medially and pull up strongly on lateral side) • Interlock stirrups with **2 horizontal strips** (strong lateral pull)	• continue with **modified basketweave** (extra pull on lateral side, particularly for vertical strip)	• for more mobility, **fanned stirrups** can be used • if sprain is limited only to this ligament horizontal strips are optional
REINFORCEMENT Ankle locks	• **2 lateral locks** (pull up strongly on lateral side)	• **2 lateral locks** (extra pull on lateral side) • **1 medial lock** (with less tension)	• continue with **2 lateral** and **1 medial** locks or • if tight boots are necessary, **1 lateral** lock plus **1 V-lock** replaces second lateral lock (V-lock with extra pull on horizontal part and final lateral vertical strip)
STABILIZATION Figure 8 variations	• **simple figure 8** (start medially and pull up strongly on lateral side)	• **heel locking figure 8** for added stability (always pull up strongly on lateral side)	• continue with **heel locking figure 8** or • if more plantar flexion needed for sport, use reverse figure 8 (ensure that end-range plantar flexion is limited with previous locking strips or with closing figure 8) • if tight, rigid boots are necessary, omit this step
CLOSING UP:	• add **felt heel-lift** for weightbearing	• **heel-lift** (optional)	**Purpose:** • *supports* calcaneo-fibular ligament • *prevents* inversion • *limits* end-range eversion and extreme plantar flexion • *permits* functional plantar flexion

TIP:
Visualize location and direction of ligament being supported during tape application.

6

ANATOMICAL AREA: FOOT AND ANKLE

INJURY: CALCANEO-FIBULAR LIGAMENT SPRAIN

T ERMINOLOGY
- middle third of the lateral ankle ligamentous complex
- long, strong, cordlike band
- from tip of fibula inferiorly, and posteriorly to lateral tubercle on the calcaneus
- see **anatomy illustration**, p. 55

E TIOLOGY
- a medial force on the lower leg when a dorsiflexed foot is relatively fixed in or forced into inversion
- more often sprained than medial side due to:
  a. a thinner, weaker less continuous ligamentous complex
  b. medial malleolus, being higher, offers less stability, allowing the talus to rock medially when stressed
- most frequently injured in combination with the anterior talo-fibular ligament

S YMPTOMS
- local pain, swelling and discolouration
- tenderness on lateral side of ankle inferior and slightly posterior to the tip of the malleolus
- active movement testing: pain on inversion
- passive movement testing: pain on inversion
- resistance testing (neutral position): no significant pattern of pain on moderate resistance
- stress testing:
  a. pain with or without some laxity on talar tilt test indicates a 1st- or 2nd-degree sprain
  b. instability or 'opening up' on the talar tilt test (often with little or no pain) can be indicative of a 3rd-degree sprain of this ligament

T REATMENT
Early
- R.I.C.E.S.
- taping: first 48 hours: **Acute Ankle Injury (open basketweave)** (p. 76)
- therapeutic modalities
Later
- continued therapy including:
  a. therapeutic modalities
  b. transverse friction massage
  c. modified fitness activities
- progressive pain-free rehabilitation including:
  a. range of motion
  b. flexibility
  c. strength: non-weight bearing to weight bearing (endurance, then power)
  d. proprioception
- gradual reintegration to sports activity with specific taped support. **See Ankle Rehabilitation taping for isolated fibulo-calcaneal ligament sprain: p. 105 (when injured in combination with anterior talo-fibular ligament, refer to taping for lateral ankle sprain, rehabilitation stage: p. 82**
- prevention of recurrence of injury

S EQUELAE
- lateral instability if ligament is not supported in a shortened position during the healing phase
- peroneal strain often accompanies this sprain, predisposing to persistent weakness and/or tendinitis of peroneal muscles
- reduced proprioception
- recurrent sprains
- chronic swelling inferior and posterior to tip of lateral malleolus
- arthritic changes

R.I.C.E.S.: Rest, Ice, Compress, Elevate, Support

SPECIFIC ANKLE REHABILITATION TAPING FOR ISOLATED POSTERIOR TALO-FIBULAR LIGAMENT SPRAIN

Positioning: seated, with the calf supported and the foot held at a 90 degree angle **BASIC STRIPS**	PROGRESSIVE STRIP ADAPTATIONS		
	SUB-ACUTE: (beginning to weightbear) • activity depends on stage of healing • how much swelling? • weightbearing only if no pain!	FUNCTIONAL: (moderate to dynamic activity) • adequate support for individual ligament • enough mobility for moderate activity	RETURN TO SPORT: (training, then competition) • reinforced support • adaptations for specific needs of sport
BASIC PREPARATION (clean, shave, spray) underwrap anchors	• if swelling is likely, use a **felt 'J'**-lateral side (bevel the edges)	• if swelling persists, continue with **felt 'J'** • for increasing activity use **heel and lace pads**	• **use heel and lace pads**
LATERAL SUPPORT Stirrups	**modified basketweave** composed of: • **3 stirrups (vertical)** (start medially and pull up strongly on lateral side) • Interlock stirrups with **2 horizontal strips** (strong lateral pull)	• continue with **modified basketweave** (extra pull on lateral side, particularly for vertical strips)	• continue with **modified basketweave** (extra pull, particularly on lateral horizontal strips) • for more mobility, **fanned stirrups** can be used
REINFORCEMENT Ankle locks	• **2 lateral locks** (pull up strongly on lateral side)	• **2 lateral locks** (extra pull on lateral side) • **1 medial lock** (with less tension)	• continue with **2 lateral** and **1 medial** locks *or* • if tight boots are necessary, **1 lateral** lock plus **1 V-lock** replaces second lateral lock (V-lock with extra pull on horizontal part and final lateral vertical strip)
STABILIZATION Figure 8 variations	• **simple figure 8** (start medially and pull up strongly on lateral side)	• **heel locking figure 8** for added stability (always pull up strongly on lateral side)	• continue with **heel locking figure 8** *or* • if injury was caused by extreme dorsiflexion or if more plantar flexion needed for sport, use **reverse figure 8** • if tight, rigid boots are necessary, omit this step
CLOSING UP:	• add **felt heel-lift** for weightbearing	• continue using **heel-lift**	**Purpose:** • *supports* posterior talo-fibular ligament • *prevents* inversion • *limits* dorsiflexion and lateral rotation of foot • *permits* functional plantar flexion

TIP:
Visualize location and direction of ligament being supported during tape application.

ANATOMICAL AREA: FOOT AND ANKLE

INJURY: POSTERIOR TALO-FIBULAR LIGAMENT SPRAIN

T ERMINOLOGY
- posterior band of the lateral ligamentous complex
- deep, thick fibres
- from the posterior aspect of the malleolus to the posterior-lateral tubercle of the talus
- see **anatomy illustration**, p. 55

E TIOLOGY
- extreme forced dorsiflexion
- weight-bearing plantarflexion with stressed external rotation of the foot
- rare as an isolated tear
- usually only ruptured in severe sprains or dislocations
- pole vaulters, parachute jumpers and ice hockey players (high-speed impact with boards) are prone to this injury

S YMPTOMS
- local pain, swelling and discolouration
- tenderness posterior to the lateral malleous deep into the peroneal tendons
- active movement testing: pain on end-range dorsiflexion possible
- passive movement testing: posterio-lateral pain on end-range dorsiflexion
- resistance testing (neutral position): no significant pattern of pain on moderate resistance
- stress testing:
  a. posterolateral pain often can be felt when stressing the deltoid ligament on the medial side (eversion of the calcaneus causes simultaneous pinching and compression of the injured ligament)
  b. pain, with or without laxity, on the 'posterior drawer' test (backward gliding of the talus under the tibia), worse with outward rotation of the foot, indicates a 1st- or 2nd-degree sprain
  c. instability (the fibula slides forward and the head of the talus moves laterally) on backward displacement of the talus, with or without pain, indicates a possible 3rd-degree sprain

R.I.C.E.S.: Rest, Ice, Compress, Elevate, Support

T REATMENT
Early
- R.I.C.E.S.
- taping: first 48 hours: **Acute Ankle Injury (open basketweave)** (p. 76)
- therapeutic modalities
Later
- Continued therapy including:
  a. therapeutic modalities
  b. transverse friction massage (this ligament is difficult to access: deep in the peroneal tendons)
  c. modified fitness activities
- progressive pain-free rehabilitation:
  a. range of motion
  b. flexibility
  c. strength: non-weight bearing to weight bearing (endurance, then power)
  d. proprioception
- gradual pain-free reintegration to sports activity with specific taping. **See Ankle rehabilitation taping for isolated posterior talo-fibular sprains, p. 107**
- prevention of further sprains

S EQUELAE
- lateral instability if ligament is not supported in a shortened position during the healing phase
- weakness of ankle musculature
- reduced proprioception
- peroneal weakness and/or tendinitis

SPECIFIC ANKLE REHABILITATION TAPING FOR ISOLATED DELTOID LIGAMENT SPRAIN

Positioning: seated, with the calf supported and the foot held at a 90 degree angle BASIC STRIPS	PROGRESSIVE STRIP ADAPTATIONS		
	SUB-ACUTE: (beginning to weightbear) • activity depends on stage of healing • how much swelling? • weightbearing only if no pain!	FUNCTIONAL: (moderate to dynamic activity) • adequate support for individual ligament • enough mobility for moderate activity	RETURN TO SPORT: (training, then competition) • reinforced support • adaptations for specific needs of sport
BASIC PREPARATION (clean, shave, spray) underwrap anchors	• if swelling is likely, use a **felt horseshoe**-medial side (bevel the edges)	• if swelling persists, continue with **felt horseshoe** • for increasing activity use **heel and lace pads**	• **use heel and lace pads**
LATERAL SUPPORT Stirrups	**modified basketweave** composed of: • **3 stirrups (vertical)** (start laterally and pull up strongly on medial side) • Interlock stirrups with **2 horizontal strips**	• continue with **modified basketweave** (extra pull on medial side, for both horizontal and vertical strips)	• continue with **modified basketweave** (extra pull, particularly on medial side) • for more mobility, **fanned stirrups** can be used
REINFORCEMENT Ankle locks	• **2 medial locks** (pull up strongly on lateral side)	• **2 medial locks** (extra pull on lateral side) • **1 lateral lock** (with less tension)	• if tight boots are necessary, **1 medial lock** plus **1 V-lock** replaces second medial lock (V-lock with main tension pulling up on last component posterior vertical strip) • **1 lateral V-lock** replaces the lateral lock (with main tension pulling up from behind heel and across anteriorly: horizontal component)
STABILIZATION Figure 8 variations	• **simple figure 8** (start tape medial to lateral and pull up strongly on medial side)	• if anterior fibres are involved, use a **heel-locking figure 8** (with medial support) *or* • if posterior fibres are involved, use a **reverse figure 8** (with medial support) (to support medial side, start tape from medial to lateral and always pull up strongly on the medial side)	• continue with **medial heel-locking figure 8** *or* • if more plantar flexion is needed for sport, or posterior fibers are involved, use **reverse figure 8** (supporting medial side) • if tight, rigid boots are necessary, omit this step
CLOSING UP:	• add **felt heel-lift** for weightbearing	• when posterior fibres are involved, continue to use **heel-lift**	**Purpose:** • *supports* medial collateral ligament complex • *prevents* eversion • *limits* dorsiflexion and lateral flexion • *limits* end-range inversion and extreme flexion • *permits* functional plantar flexion

TIP:
Visualize location and direction of ligament being supported during tape application.

ANATOMICAL AREA: FOOT AND ANKLE

INJURY: DELTOID LIGAMENT SPRAIN

T ERMINOLOGY
- medial lateral ligamentous complex
- superficial and deep portions
- from the medial malleolus anteriorly to the navicular (superficial) and to the talus (deep), inferiorly to the calcaneus and posteriorly to the talus (both superficial and deep fibres)
- see **anatomy illustration**, p. 54

E TIOLOGY
- a lateral force on the lower leg when foot is relatively fixed in extension
- less often sprained than lateral complex due to:
  a. thicker, stronger, more continuous ligament fibres
  b. lateral malleolus being lower offers more stability to medial side by preventing a lateral talar tilt
- occurs in wrestlers and parachute jumpers

S YMPTOMS
- local pain, swelling and discolouration
- locations of tenderness around medial malleolus is indicative of injury site
- active movement testing: pain on eversion
- passive movement testing: pain on eversion
- resistance testing (neutral position): no significant pattern of pain on moderate resistance
- stress testing:
  a. medial pain with or without some laxity on talar tilt test in 1st- and 2nd-degree sprains
  b. anterior pain with or without some laxity on anterior drawer test is indicative of injury to the anterior fibres – 1st- and 2nd-degree sprains
  c. posterior pain with or without some laxity on posterior drawer test is indicative of damage to the posterior fibres – 1st- and 2nd-degree sprains
  d. complete instability on any of the above three tests is indicative of a possible 3rd-degree sprain which is often less painful than 2nd degree

R.I.C.E.S. : Rest, Ice, Compress, Elevate, Support

T REATMENT
Early
  R.I.C.E.S.
- taping: first 48 hours: **Acute Ankle Injury (open basketweave with medial reinforcement)** (p. 76)
- therapeutic modalities
Later
- continued therapy including:
  a. therapeutic modalities
  b. transverse friction massage
- modified fitness activities
- progressive pain-free rehabilitation including:
  a. range of motion
  b. flexibility
  c. strength: non-weight bearing to weight bearing (endurance, then power)
  d. proprioception
- gradual pain-free reintegration to sports activity with specific taping. **See Rehabilitation taping for isolated deltoid ligament sprain, p. 109**
- prevention of recurrent sprains

S EQUELAE
- medial instability if ligament is not supported in a shortened position during the healing phase
- reduced proprioception
- weakness of ankle musculature
- longer healing time
- tibialis anterior tendinitis or associated strain

SPECIFIC ANKLE REHABILITATION TAPING FOR ISOLATED ANTERIOR INFERIOR TIBIO-FIBULAR LIGAMENT SPRAIN

Positioning: seated, with the calf supported and the foot held at 10 degrees of plantar flexion **BASIC STRIPS**	PROGRESSIVE STRIP ADAPTATIONS		
	SUB-ACUTE: (beginning to weightbear) • activity depends on stage of healing • how much swelling? • weightbearing only if no pain!	FUNCTIONAL: (moderate to dynamic activity) • adequate support for individual ligament • enough mobility for moderate activity	RETURN TO SPORT: (training, then competition) • reinforced support • adaptations for specific needs of sport
BASIC PREPARATION (clean, shave, spray) underwrap anchors	• if swelling is likely, use a **felt horseshoe**-lateral side (bevel the edges)	• if swelling persists, continue with **felt horseshoe** • for increasing activity use **heel and lace pads**	• **use heel and lace pads**
LATERAL SUPPORT Stirrups	**modified basketweave** composed of: • **3 stirrups (vertical)** (start under foot and pull up equally on both sides) • Interlock stirrups with **2 horizontal strips**	• continue with **modified basketweave** (extra pull on medial side for horizontal strips)	• continue with **modified basketweave** (ensure foot is held in slight plantar flexion) • if much plantar flexion is needed for sport, **fanned stirrups** can be used
REINFORCEMENT Ankle locks	• **1 lateral V-lock** (extra pull on horizontal part and final lateral vertical strip)	• **1 lateral V-lock** (extra pull on horizontal part and final lateral vertical strip) • **1 medial V-lock** (extra pull on final vertical strip)	• continue as before with **1 lateral V-lock** plus **1 medial V-lock**
STABILIZATION Figure 8 variations	• **simple figure 8** (ensure that extreme plantar flexion is restricted with this strip)	• **reverse figure 8** (for added stability and prevention of dorsiflexion) (extra pull when crossing heel both laterally and medially)	• continue with **reverse figure 8** (ensure that end-range plantar flexion is limited with previous locking strips or with closing figure 8) • if tight, rigid boots are necessary, omit this step
CLOSING UP:	• initially add 1.5 cm (3.4 in) thick **felt heel-lift** for weightbearing to avoid dorsiflexion	• **heel-lift** imperative	**Purpose:** • *supports* medial collateral ligament complex • *prevents* eversion • *limits* dorsiflexion and lateral flexion • *limits* end-range inversion and extreme flexion • *permits* functional plantar flexion Note: this taping does not directly reinforce the fibers of the injured ligament, but reduces the stresses caused by extremes of motion

TIP:
Visualize location and direction of ligament being supported during tape application.

6

Foot and Ankle

ANATOMICAL AREA: FOOT AND ANKLE

INJURY: ANTERIOR INFERIOR TIBIO-FIBULAR LIGAMENT SPRAIN

T ERMINOLOGY

- anterior aspect of the ligamentous mortice of the talo-crural joint (ankle proper) running from the anterolateral border of the tibia to the anteromedial border of the fibula meeting just superior to the talus. This ligament is thinner and weaker than its counterpart, the posterior inferior tibio-fibular ligament
- see **anatomy illustration**, p. 55

E TIOLOGY

- stressed in full dorsiflexion: the wider aspect of the talus jams between the malleoli
- stressed severely when a dorsiflexed foot is rotated laterally, forcing the malleoli to separate
- can be accompanied by posterior fibulo-calcaneal ligament sprain
- common injury in competitive alpine skiing

S YMPTOMS

- local pain, swelling and discolouration
- tenderness anteriorly on palpation between the tibia and fibula just superior to the talus
- active movement testing: pain on dorsiflexion at end-range; increased with active eversion
- passive movement testing: pain on dorsiflexion at end-range
- resistance testing (neutral position): no significant pattern of pain on moderate resistance
- stress testing:
  a. palpable displacement when squeezing malleoli together (may be accompanied by pain from pinching of ligament fibres)
  b. marked diastasis (opening up) of malleoli on forced varus in 3rd-degree sprains
  c. in chronic cases, there is often an audible click on forced varus into an excessive range

T REATMENT

Early

- R.I.C.E.S.
- taping: first 48 hours: **Acute Ankle Injury (open basketweave – position with slight plantarflexion)**
- therapeutic modalities

Later:

- continued therapy including:
  a. therapeutic modalities
  b. transverse friction massage
- modified fitness activities
- progressive pain-free rehabilitation including:
  a. range of motion
  b. flexibility
  c. strength: non-weight bearing to weight bearing (endurance, then power)
  d. proprioception
- prevention of recurrent sprains
- gradual pain-free reintegration to sports activity with specific taping. **See rehabilitation taping for isolated anterior inferior tibio-fibular ligament sprains, p. 111**
- needs greater non-weight bearing (NWB) rehabilitation phase due to inherent displacing stress caused by weight bearing

S EQUELAE

- lateral talo-crural instability if ligament is not supported in shortened position during healing phase
- permanent instability of the ankle mortice
- dysfunction of the superior tibio-fibular joint
- peroneal strain and residual weakness often accompany this sprain
- weakness of all ankle musculature
- recurrent injury

R.I.C.E.S.: Rest, Ice, Compress, Elevate, Support

ANATOMICAL AREA: THE CALF

TAPING FOR CALF CONTUSION OR STRAIN

Purpose

- applies localized specific compression to the bruised or torn tissues (decreases subsequent swelling, bleeding and the chances of further tissue damage in the area)
- supports the calf muscles by elastic reinforcement assisting plantarflexion
- prevents full stretch of the musculo-tendinous unit by restricting dorsiflexion
- limits inversion significantly when heel lock is used
- allows full plantarflexion and eversion

Indications for use

- calf strains or contusions in muscle bulks or musculo-tendinous junctions

NOTES:

- The exact site of the contusion or strain must be localized.
- Underwrap is not recommended as it significantly lessens the effectiveness of the taping technique. If necessary, a hypoallergenic liquid such as Comfeel™ can be used instead.
- Cold packing of the area should be started immediately.

MATERIALS

Razor
Skin toughener spray/adhesive spray
7.5 cm (3 in) elastic adhesive bandage
3.8 cm (1½ in) non-elastic tape
7.5 cm (3 in) or 10 cm (4 in) elastic wrap
1.5 cm felt heel lift

For additional details regarding an injury example, see T.E.S.T.S. chart, p. 117.

Positioning

Lying prone at the end of a low bench with a folded towel placed under the thigh superior to (above) the patella and the calf extending over the end of the bench.

Procedure

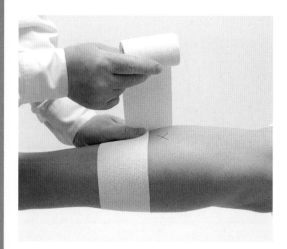

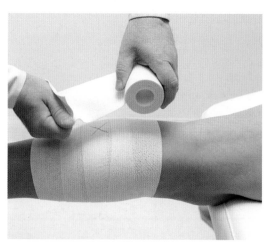

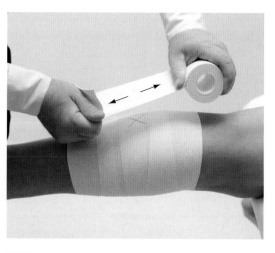

1 Make sure the area to be taped is clean and relatively hair free; shave if necessary

2 *Check skin for cuts, blisters or areas of irritation before spraying with skin toughener or spray adhesive.* Spray circumferentially to the entire calf and let dry completely.

3 Localize the exact site of the contusion or muscle strain. Beginning 7.5 cm below the lower aspect of the injury, using light tension, wrap 7.5 cm elastic adhesive tape around the limb. Repeat this strip, overlapping the previous one by 1.25 cm ($\frac{1}{2}$ in) until the entire injured area is covered and surpassed by 7.5 cm.

 NOTE:
This first layer of tape forms a foundation for the compression strips, which avoids excessive tension on the skin.

4a Prepare to apply the first pressure strip directly below the centre of the site of injury: fold back 10 cm at the end of a roll of 7.5 cm elastic adhesive tape in one hand, and hold the remainder of the roll in the other.

4b Stretch the tape fully and keep it stretched laterally.

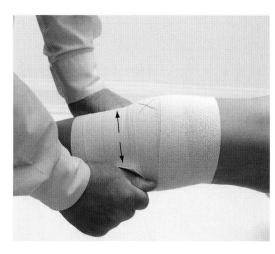

4c Apply strong pressure to the limb equally with both hands while maintaining the lateral stretch until the tape reaches three-quarters of the way around the limb.

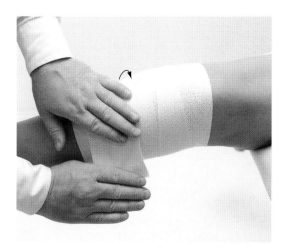

4d Being careful to keep the strip from detaching, release the tension while holding the stretched part against the limb, before adhering the tape end without any tension at all.

NOTE:

Application of this strip causes some discomfort.

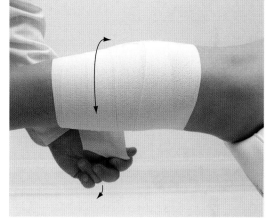

4e Finish encircling the limb with the other end of the strip in the same manner, completely overlapping the tape ends at the back.

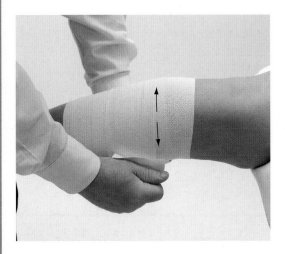

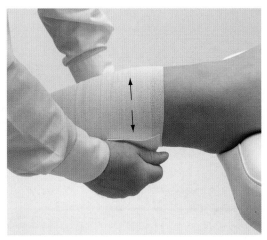

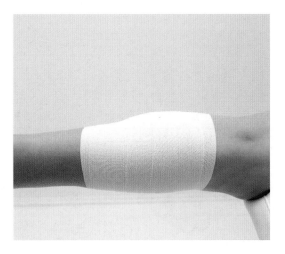

5   Repeat the pressure strip, overlapping by half the tape width above the last strip more proximally, focusing the pressure directly over the injury.

 NOTE:
This may be quite painful when pressure is applied directly over the site.

6   Continue repeating the pressure strips, moving proximally until the entire tape base is covered.

 TIP:
Ensure that the tape job extends at least one full tape-width lower and higher than the area of the injury.

NOTE:
The finished compression taping should have no wrinkles, should be neat in appearance and have continuous, localized pressure over the injured site from distal to proximal.

7   For dynamic support, use the compression taping as the proximal anchor and apply the Achilles tendon taping technique. This will protect and support the entire musculo-tendinous unit for weight-bearing activities. (See Achilles tendon taping technique, p. 118.)

6

Calf strain

ANATOMICAL AREA: CALF

INJURY: CALF STRAIN

T ERMINOLOGY
- gastrocnemius or soleus strain
- Achilles tendon complex strain: 'pulled' heel cord
- degree of severity: 1st to 3rd – see strain chart, p. 36
- torn Achilles tendon: 3rd-degree strain

E TIOLOGY
- sudden forced dorsiflexion during active plantarflexion
- explosive plantarflexion against resistance
- overstretching
- external impact to calf (contusion)
- inadequate warm-up

S YMPTOMS
- history of sudden sharp pain
- 'pop' sensation
- feeling of 'being shot' in the calf
- varying degrees of pain at injury site
- local swelling and gradual discolouration
- active movement testing:
  a. no significant pain on non-weight bearing movements
  b. calf pain on active plantarflexion if weight bearing
  c. calf pain on dorsiflexion if tight calf is being stretched
- passive movement testing: pain on dorsiflexion (1st and 2nd degrees)
- resistance testing (neutral position):
  a. pain on mild to moderate resistance and weakness of plantarflexion (1st and 2nd degrees of severity)
  b. inability to plantarflex with little or no pain is indicative of 3rd degree of severity (complete rupture)

T REATMENT
Early
- R.I.C.E.S.
- taping: **Compression Taping**
- heel lift
- therapeutic modalities
- active contraction of dorsiflexors to induce relaxation and improve flexibility of calf (isometric at first)

Later
- continued therapy including:
  a. therapeutic modalities
  b. flexibility
  c. strengthening
  d. proprioception
- rehabilitation programme: non-weight bearing initially, progressing to dynamic pain-free reintegration with taped support
- transverse friction massage (only after several weeks when scar tissue is adhering)

S EQUELAE
- scarring
- haematoma if massaged too early
- inflexibility
- weakness
- highly prone to re-straining/cramping

R.I.C.E.S.: Rest, Ice, Compress, Elevate, Support

ANATOMICAL AREA: CALF

TAPING FOR ACHILLES TENDON INJURY

Purpose

- supports the Achilles tendon with elastic reinforcement assisting plantarflexion
- prevents full stretch of the musculo-tendinous unit by restricting full dorsiflexion
- limits inversion significantly when heel lock is used
- permits full plantarflexion and eversion

Indications for use

- Achilles tendon strain
- Achilles tendinitis
- diffuse heel pain (possible bursitis)
- calf strain; use in combination with **Compression Taping**
- calf contusion: use in combination with **Compression Taping**
- peroneus longus strain or tendinitis: use in combination with **Peroneus Longus Support Strips**, p. 125
- tibialis posterior strain or tendinitis: use in combination with **Tibialis Posterior Support Strips**, p. 129

NOTES:

- Be sure that a thorough assessment of the region has been carried out prior to taping.
- If a third-degree strain is suspected, the athlete must be seen by a surgeon as soon as possible.
- Evaluate the site of injury; pain may be located at the base of the Achilles tendon, in the belly of the muscle or at the musculo-tendinous junction.
- During taping, neutral alignment of the foot can be controlled by the taper whose thigh is used to counter-pressure against the athlete's great toe.
- Because Achilles taping pulls the foot into plantarflexion, the ankle is rendered less stable and the risk of an inversion sprain is increased (step 13 demonstrates preventive measures).
- Once taped, a felt or foam heel lift in the athlete's shoe will shorten and help support the Achilles tendon by improving its mechanical advantage.

For additional details regarding an injury example see T.E.S.T.S. chart, p. 124.

> ### MATERIALS
> Razor
> Skin toughener spray/adhesive spray
> Underwrap
> 3.8 cm (1½ in) non-elastic tape
> 5 cm (2 in) elastic adhesive bandage
> 7.5 cm (3 in) elastic adhesive bandage
> 2 cm (¾ in) felt or dense foam heel lift

Position

Lying prone (face down) with the shin resting on a cushioned support and the foot protruding over the edge of the table (for steps 1–4 it is more convenient to have the subject supine with the lower limb extending over the end of the table at midcalf).

Procedure

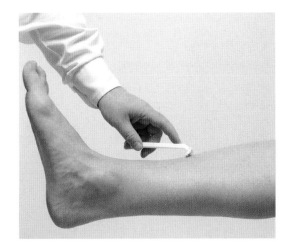

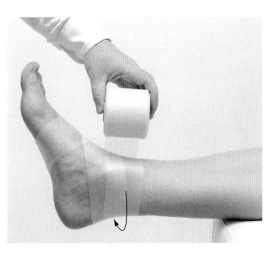

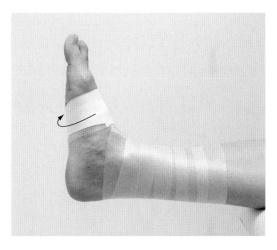

1 Make sure the area to be taped is clean and relatively hair free; shave if necessary.

2 Check skin for cuts, blisters or areas of irritation before spraying with skin toughener or spray adhesive.

3 Apply underwrap without tension around the ankle up to lower one-third of calf. **Avoid wrinkles**.

NOTE:
Heel and lace pads should be used when the taping is to assist the athlete to resume training or competition.

4 Apply two circumferential anchors of 3.8 cm non-elastic tape at the level of heads of the metatarsals.

TIP:
Be sure to allow some splaying of the metatarsals.

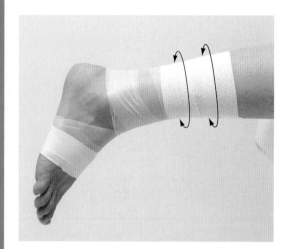 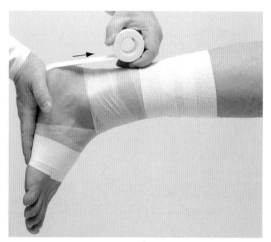 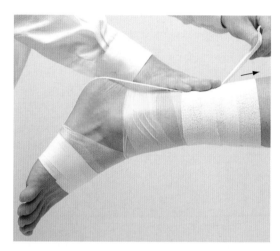

5 At this stage, ask the athlete to turn and lie prone to facilitate the rest of the taping technique. Using only slight tension, apply two circumferential anchors of 5 cm elastic adhesive bandage at the midbelly of the calf muscle.

6a **a.** Apply the first vertical strip using either 5 cm or 7.5 cm elastic adhesive bandage. Fix it firmly, **without tension**, to the plantar surface of the foot. **b.** Pull upwards from the centre of the back of the calcaneus **with strong tension** to the lower edge of the calf anchor.

6c Support this strip without loosening its tension and carefully apply the last 5 cm of tape with virtually **no tension** before cutting the tape from the roll.

 TIP:
Allow the ankle to plantarflex.

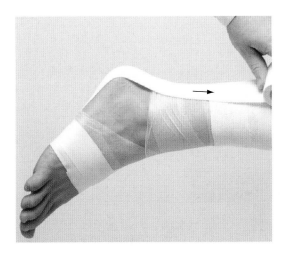

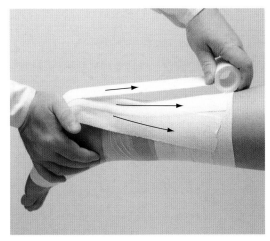

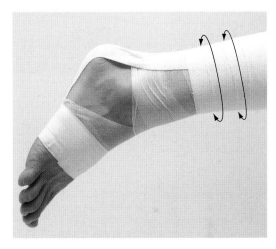

7 Repeat step 6, passing just laterally to the centre of back of heel, pulling up firmly to control the medial tilt of the calcaneus.

TIP:

Maintain strong tension while adhering the upper end of this strip to the calf anchor before cutting the tape

8 Repeat step 6, passing just medially to the centre of back of heel, controlling the lateral tilt and forming a 'V' over the Achilles tendon posteriorly before re-anchoring strips at both ends.

NOTE:

Special reinforcement strips should be added after this strip before going on to step 9.

9 Close up the calf portion of the tape job with circumferential strips of elastic adhesive tape.

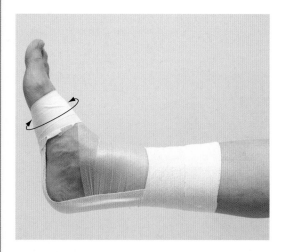

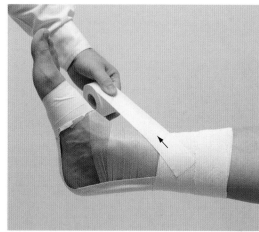

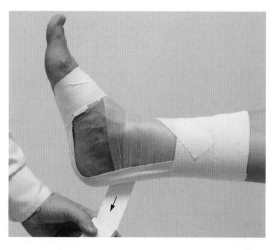

10 Reposition the athlete in the supine position to facilitate the next steps.

11 Apply non-elastic tape anchor to the midfoot over the heads of the metatarsals.

12 Close up the foot portion of the tape job with circumferential strips of non-elastic tape, overlapping each previous strip by half.

13a A lateral lock is applied to offer stability to the lateral ankle. Beginning on the medial side of the upper anchor, pass down across the anterior skin.

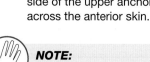

NOTE:

Once the foot is held in plantarflexion, ankle stability is compromised based on the demands of the sport and the individual's ankle stability; the use of one or two ankle locks is recommended as outlined in the following, optional, procedure (steps 13 and 14).

13b Wind the tape around behind the Achilles tendon to catch the heel from the medial side.

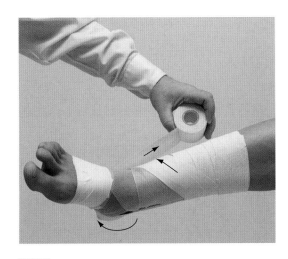

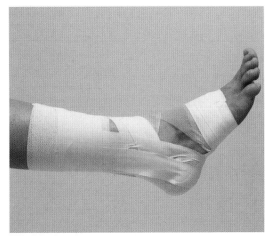

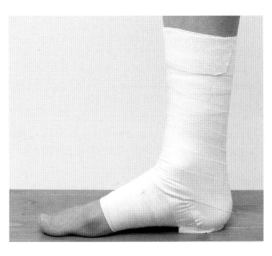

13c Lock the heel and pull the tape up with strong tension on the lateral side before affixing it to the upper anchors.

14 Repeat step 13 (a–c) a second time on the lateral side.

15 Re-anchor these locks.

 NOTE:
A medial lock can also be applied to reinforce stability in particularly vulnerable ankles.

16 Close up the entire tape job, covering any open areas.

17 Test limits of taping restriction to ensure adequate pain-free support. Dorsiflexion must be limited by at least 30°. There should be no pain on passive dorsiflexion.

18 For the acute and subacute stages cut a 2 cm felt heel lift, bevelled at the anterior (front) edge, and place it under the heel to raise it, thereby reducing tension on the tendon.

 TIP:
It is best to add heel lifts to both feet for a balanced gait.

ANATOMICAL AREA: CALF

INJURY: ACHILLES TENDINITIS

T ERMINOLOGY
- Achilles tendon inflammation (irritation)
- chronic heel cord strain

E TIOLOGY
- structural strain from repeated quick push-offs as in repetitive running
- sudden change in training; increased distance, speed or intensity; change of terrain (example: hills vs level ground)
- new footwear: inadequate heel support
- inadequate warm-up and stretching
- subsequent to a gastrocnemius (calf) strain

S YMPTOMS
- tenderness plus swelling around tendon
- localized pain (usually mid-tendon) spreads as condition progresses
- acute posterior heel pain on weight-bearing plantarflexion (particularly after resting)
- active motion testing: possible pain on plantarflexion
- passive movement testing: usually painful on dorsiflexion
- resistance testing (neutral position): possible weakness and marked pain on moderate resistance

T REATMENT
- therapy including:
   a. ice
   b. therapeutic modalities
   c. transverse friction massage
- **Achilles tendon taping,** p. 118
- heel lift
- modified training programme
- total rehabilitation programme with emphasis on full flexibility, eccentric strengthening through range of motion and dynamic proprioception
- progressive reintegration to regular sports activity with taped support as above

S EQUELAE
- persistent pain
- scarring/thickening of tendon
- inflexibility
- weakness of calf
- imbalance of ankle musculature flexibility and/or strength
- bursitis
- calcification of tendon or bursa

ANATOMICAL AREA: CALF

TAPING FOR: PERONEUS LONGUS TENDON INJURY

Purpose

- supports peroneus longus tendon with elastic reinforcement assisting plantarflexion with eversion
- prevents full stretch of the musculo-tendinous unit by restricting dorsiflexion and inversion
- permits full plantarflexion plus eversion

Indications for use

- peroneus longus tendon strain
- peroneus longus tendonitis

NOTES:

- Be sure that a thorough assessment of the region has been carried out prior to taping.
- IF A THIRD-DEGREE STRAIN IS SUSPECTED, THE ATHLETE MUST BE SEEN BY A SURGEON AS SOON AS POSSIBLE.

MATERIALS

Razor
Skin toughener spray/adhesive spray
Underwrap
5 cm (2 in) elastic adhesive bandage
7.5 cm (3 in) elastic adhesive bandage
2 cm (¾ in) felt or dense foam heel lift
3.8 cm (1.5 in) non-elastic tape

For additional details regarding an injury example see T.E.S.T.S. chart, p. 128.

Positioning

Lying supine (face up) to start, then prone (face down) with the shin resting on a cushioned support and the foot protruding over the edge of the table.

Procedure

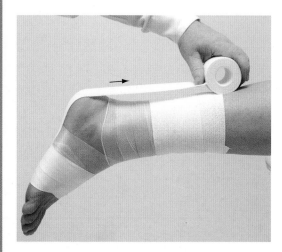

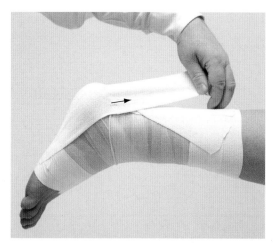

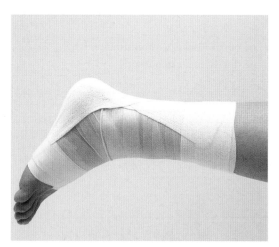

1   Begin taping by applying steps 1–8 of **Achilles tendon taping**, p. 118

NOTE:
Strips must be re-anchored before proceeding.

2a   Affix, without tension, a strip of 5 cm (2 in) elastic adhesive bandage to the plantar surface of the foot, starting on the medial side and leading diagonally across to the lateral side of the heel.

2b   Holding the foot in plantarflexion and significant eversion, pull the tape up strongly across the lateral side of the heel.

TIP:
Following the direct line of pull of this tendon.

2c   Maintain strong tension and affix the tape to the calf anchors.

TIP:
Apply the last 5 cm (2 in) of tape with no tension before cutting tape from roll.

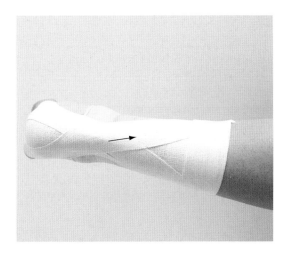

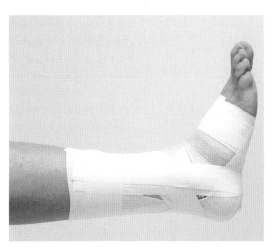

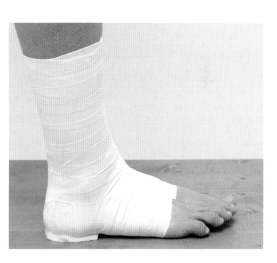

3 Repeat strip 2a–2c a second time, slightly more anterior (1 cm).

4 Continue the tape job with the **Achilles taping technique** (lateral heel-locking reinforcement is less critical in this tape job because the ankle is already pulled into eversion).

5 Test limits of taping restriction to ensure adequate pain-free support. **a**. Dorsiflexion with inversion must be restricted by at least 30°. **b**. There should be no pain on passive dorsiflexion with inversion.

TIP:
Use a heel lift to reduce the strain on the tendon when weight bearing.

ANATOMICAL AREA: CALF

INJURY: PERONEUS LONGUS TENDINITIS

T ERMINOLOGY
- chronic overuse syndrome of peroneus longus
- tenosynovitis (inflammation of tendon and sheath)

E TIOLOGY
- poor foot biomechanics (more common with high arches)
- weakness and/or inflexibility of lateral ankle muscles
- chronic overstretch or overuse
- subsequent to peroneus longus strain or chronic ankle sprains
- inadequate foot support
- repeated running on hard surfaces
- sudden change in terrain, speed, intensity, frequency, resistance, etc.
- uncommon incidence: seen in figure skaters

S YMPTOMS
- swelling and cramping
- localized thickening and tenderness of tendon
- localized heat and redness along tendon possible
- crepitation
- active movement testing:
    a. weight-bearing: pain on plantarflexion particularly if associated with eversion
    b. non-weight bearing: possible pain on plantarflexion with eversion
    c. localized pain during active dorsiflexion with inversion (if tight peroneus is being stretched)
- passive movement testing: pain on dorsiflexion with inversion (1st- and 2nd-degree sprains)
- resistance testing (neutral position): pain with or without weakness on eversion with plantarflexion

T REATMENT
- therapy including:
    a. ice
    b. therapeutic modalities
    c. transverse friction massage
- modified activity initially
- taping **for Peroneus Longus adaptation of Achilles Tendon Taping**
- selective strengthening of peroneus longus; non-weight bearing initially, progressing gradually to eccentric full weight bearing
- flexibility then strengthening of all ankle musculature
- thorough biomechanical assessment and re-education
- orthotics may be indicated
- gradual (pain-free) reintegration to sports activities with taped support as above
- total rehabilitation: progressive exercise programme for flexibility, strength and dynamic proprioception

S EQUELAE
- scarring
- inflexibility
- weakness of evertors
- muscle imbalance
- chronic tendinitis
- chronic subluxing or dislocating of tendons
- predisposition to ankle sprains
- lateral compartment syndrome

NOTE:
Inability to evert in plantarflexion with little or no pain can be indicative of a 3rd-degree strain – tendon rupture.

ANATOMICAL AREA: CALF

TAPING FOR: TIBIALIS POSTERIOR TENDON INJURY

Purpose

- supports tibialis posterior tendon with elastic reinforcement assisting plantarflexion with inversion
- prevents full stretch of the musculo-tendinous unit by restricting dorsiflexion and eversion
- limits inversion significantly when heel lock is used
- permits full plantarflexion

Indications for use

- tibialis posterior tendon strain
- tibialis posterior tendinitis

NOTES:

- Be sure that a thorough assessment of the region has been carried out prior to taping.
- IF A THIRD-DEGREE STRAIN IS SUSPECTED, THE ATHLETE MUST BE SEEN BY A SURGEON AS SOON AS POSSIBLE.

MATERIALS

Razor
Skin toughener spray/spray adhesive
Underwrap
5 cm (2 in) elastic adhesive tape
7.5 cm (3 in) elastic adhesive tape
2 cm (¾ in) felt or dense foam heel lift
3.8 cm (1½ in) white tape

For additional details regarding an injury example see T.E.S.T.S. chart, p. 132.

Positioning

Lying supine (face up) to start with, then lying prone (face down) with the shin resting on a cushioned support and the foot protruding over the edge of the table.

Procedure

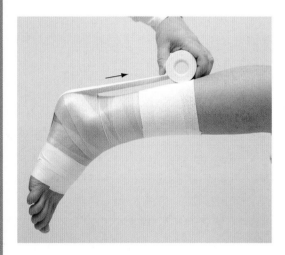

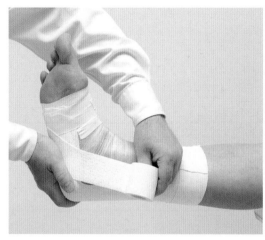

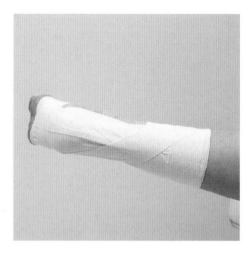

1   Begin taping by applying steps 1–8 of **Achilles tendon taping**, p. 118.

NOTE:
Re-anchor strips before proceeding.

2a   Affix, without tension, a strip of 5 cm (2 in) elastic adhesive tape to the plantar surface of the foot, starting on the lateral side and leading diagonally across to the medial side of the heel.

2b   Holding the foot in plantarflexion and significant inversion, pull the tape up strongly across the medial side of the heel.

TIP:
Following the direct line of pull of the posterior tibialis tendon.

2c   Maintain strong tension and affix the tape to the calf anchors.

TIP:
Apply the last 5 cm of tape with no tension before cutting.

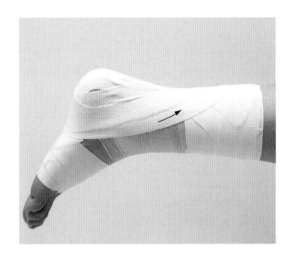

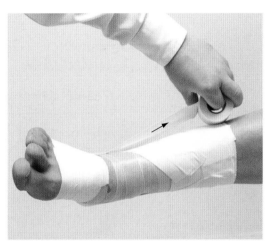

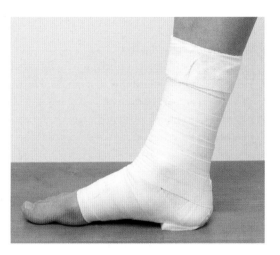

3 Repeat strip 2a–2c a second time, slightly more anterior (1 cm).

4 Continue the tape job with the **Achilles taping**, p. 118.

 NOTE:
It is essential to reinforce lateral ligament structures with a heel lock to prevent inversion.

5 Test limits of taping restriction to ensure adequate pain-free support. **a**. Dorsiflexion with eversion must be limited by at least 30° or more. **b**. There should be no pain on passive dorsiflexion with eversion.

 TIP:
Use a heel lift to reduce the strain on the tendon when weight bearing.

6

Foot and Ankle

ANATOMICAL AREA: CALF

INJURY: TIBIALIS POSTERIOR TENDINITIS

T ERMINOLOGY
- chronic overuse syndrome of tibialis posterior
- shin splints
- tenosynovitis (inflammation of tendon and sheath)

E TIOLOGY
- overly pronated or flat feet
- poor foot biomechanics (a fixed forefoot inversion with a valgus calcaneus)
- weakness and/or inflexibility of medial ankle muscles
- chronic overstretch or overuse
- subsequent to tibialis posterior strain or chronic ankle sprains
- inadequate foot support
- repeated running on hard surfaces
- sudden change in terrain, speed, intensity, frequency, resistance, etc.
- common in joggers and ballet dancers

S YMPTOMS
- pain posterior to medial malleolus extending up to posteromedial border of tibia (can radiate down to the medial arch)
- localized swelling and thickening of tendon
- exquisitely tender on palpation of inflamed site
- local heat and redness over tendon possible
- crepitation
- active movement testing:
  a. weight bearing: pain, particularly at push-off
  b. non-weight bearing: possible pain on plantarflexion with inversion
  c. pain on dorsiflexion with eversion
- passive movement testing: pain on dorsiflexion with eversion
- resistance testing (neutral position): pain with or without weakness on resisted inversion with plantarflexion

NOTE:
Inability to invert in plantarflexion with little or no pain can indicate a 3rd-degree strain – tendon rupture.

T REATMENT
- therapy including:
  a. ice
  b. therapeutic modalities (laser or ultrasound can be particularly helpful)
  c. transverse friction massage
- modified activity initially
- taping **for Tibialis Posterior adaptation of Achilles Tendon taping**, p. 118
- selective strengthening of tibialis posterior; non-weight bearing initially, progressing to eccentric full weight bearing
- strengthening and flexibility of all ankle musculature
- thorough biomechanical assessment and re-education
- orthotics may be indicated
- gradual pain-free reintegration programme with taped support as above
- total rehabilitation: progressive exercise programme for flexibility, strength and dynamic proprioception

S EQUELAE
- scarring
- inflexibility
- weakness of invertors
- muscle imbalance
- chronic tendinitis
- chronic shin splints
- deep posterior compartment syndrome (surgical splitting of fascia sometimes necessary in severe cases)
- predisposition to stress fractures

Chapter 7 KNEE AND THIGH

The knee is a modified, hinged weight-bearing joint dependent on several structures for stability:

- **medial and lateral collateral ligaments** to prevent lateral (sideways) shearing movements
- **anterior and posterior cruciate ligaments** to prevent anterior (forward) and posterior (backwards) displacement during movement
- **menisci (two wedge-shaped cartilages)** form mechanical spacers to cushion forces, guide movements and add to overall stability.

The patella, while improving the biomechanical efficiency of the quadriceps and protecting the femoral condyles, can often be a source of knee pain.

The knee is frequently injured during sporting activity, especially contact sports, due to several factors:

- heavy weight-bearing demands on the knee during sporting activities
- mechanical disadvantages at extremes of performance, e.g. a relatively weak medial collateral ligament and its attachment to the medial meniscus
- extremes of force as seen in tackling that can lead to severe injuries such as anterior cruciate ligament ruptures.

Correct taping and treatment for knee problems allow the athlete to continue sports participation with minimal risk of sustaining further injury. Taped support assists stability to the injured structure, enhances end-range proprioceptive feedback, and promotes healing by allowing dynamic function.

Knee and Thigh

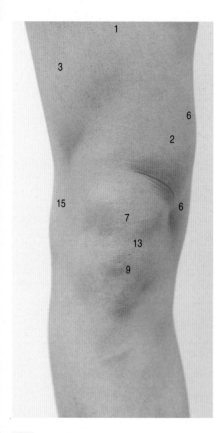

1   Anterior knee.

Behind the knee on the lateral side, the rounded tendon of biceps femoris (12) can be felt easily, with the broad, strap-like iliotibial tract (17) in front of it, with a furrow between them. On the medial side, two tendons can be felt: the narrow rounded semitendinosus (14) just behind the broader semimembranosus (5). At the front, the patellar ligament (13) keeps the patella (7) at a constant distance from the tibial tuberosity (9), while at the side the adjacent margin of the femoral condyle and tibial plateau can be palpated.

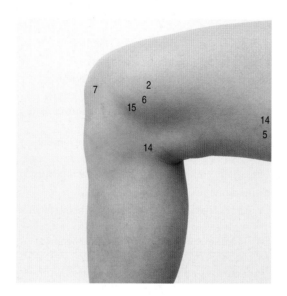

2   Medial knee.

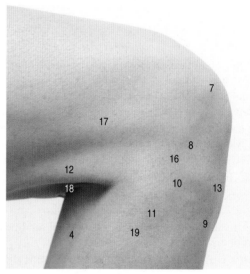

3   Lateral knee.

MUSCLES

1. Quadriceps: rectus femoris
2. Quadriceps: vastus medialis
3. Quadriceps: vastus lateralis
4. Gastrocnemius
5. Semimembranosus
6. Adductor magnus

BONES

7. Patella
8. Margin of lateral condyle of femur
9. Tibial tuberosity
10. Margin of tibial plateau
11. Head of fibula

TENDONS AND LIGAMENTS

12. Biceps femoris

13. Patellar tendon/ligament
14. Semitendinosus
15. Medial collateral ligament
16. Lateral collateral ligament

FASCIA

17. Iliotibial tract

HOLLOWS

18. Popliteal fossa

NERVES

19. Common peroneal

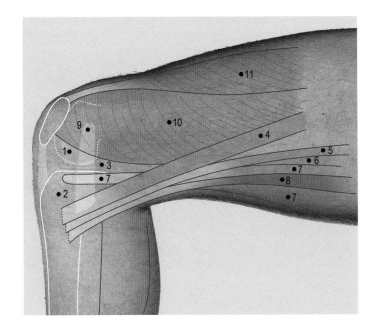

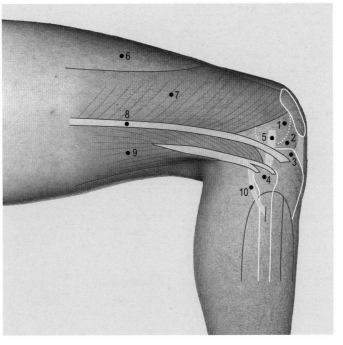

MEDIAL ASPECT OF THE FLEXED KNEE: BONES AND MUSCLES

1. Medial femoral condyle
2. Medial tibial condyle
3. Medial meniscus
4. Sartorius
5. Gracilis
6. Adductor magnus
7. Semimembranosus
8. Semitendinosus
9. Medial collateral ligament
10. Vastus medialis
11. Rectus femoris

LATERAL ASPECT OF THE FLEXED KNEE: BONES AND SOFT TISSUES

1. Lateral femoral condyle
2. Lateral meniscus
3. Lateral tibial condyle
4. Head of fibula
5. Lateral collateral ligament
6. Rectus femoris
7. Vastus lateralis
8. Iliotibial tract
9. Biceps femoris
10. Common peroneal nerve

ANATOMICAL AREA: KNEE AND THIGH

TAPING FOR MEDIAL COLLATERAL LIGAMENT KNEE SPRAIN

Purpose

- supports the medial collateral ligament (MCL) by tightening the medial aspect of the joint line
- prevents the last 15° of knee extension and external rotation of the tibia under the femur
- allows almost full flexion and functional extension of the knee

Indications for use

- MCL sprains: 1st and 2nd degree
- post immobilization of 3rd-degree MCL sprains
- for medial meniscus injuries: emphasize spiral strips which cause internal rotation of the tibia

MATERIALS

Razor
Skin toughener spray/adhesive spray
Underwrap
7.5 cm (3 in) and 10 cm (4 in) elastic adhesive bandage
5 cm (2 in) and 3.8 cm (1½ in) non-elastic tape
15.2 cm (6 in) elastic wrap
Skin lubricant
Heel and lace pads

NOTES:

- Ensure that the correct diagnosis has been made. **If in doubt, refer!**
- Always assess which knee and which side of that knee was injured (the athlete may have sustained spraining on the medial aspect and bruising on the lateral aspect of the same knee).
- During exercise, increased blood circulation causes swelling of thigh muscles. Ensure that circumferential strips are affixed with only light tension, avoiding constriction and possible cramping of thigh and calf muscles.
- Avoid taping over the patella, as this can cause compression, pain and subsequent problems.

For additional details regarding an injury example see T.E.S.T.S. chart, p. 144.

Positioning

Standing upright. Place a roll of tape under the heel of the foot of the injured knee, so that the knee is slightly flexed. The foot is turned inwards to medially rotate the tibia under the femur (releasing the tension from the MCL). Eighty percent of the body weight should be supported by the uninjured side.

TIP:
For stability, have the athlete lean against a wall or couch (plinth) for support.

Procedure

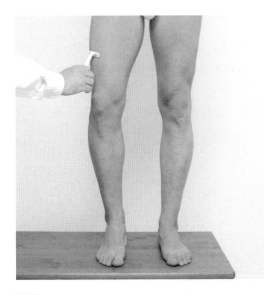

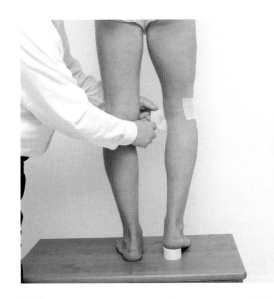

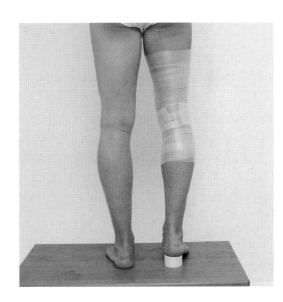

1 Make sure the area to be taped is clean and relatively hair free; shave if necessary.

2 Check skin for cuts, blisters or areas of irritation before spraying with skin toughener or spray adhesive.

3 Place lubricated pads over the hamstring tendons.

4 Spray midthigh and midcalf with skin toughener or adhesive spray.

5 Apply underwrap from midthigh to midcalf.

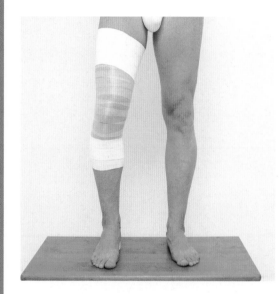

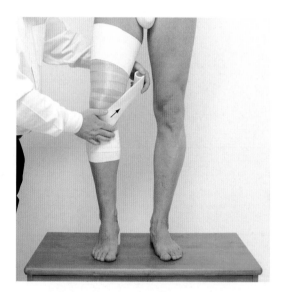

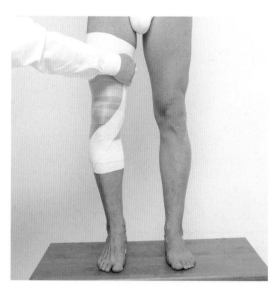

6 Apply 2 circumferential anchors of 10 cm elastic adhesive bandage, using only slight tension, to the midthigh and midcalf regions, covering the skin well beyond the edge of the underwrap.

 NOTE:
Re-check the athlete's position.

7 Place a strip of 7.5 cm elastic adhesive bandage starting from the posteromedial aspect of the distal anchor, spiralling around the lateral side of the tibia, anteriorly. Cross medially below the patella with moderate tension and pull proximally with strong tension over the medial joint line to the proximal anchor.

 NOTE:
This strip helps to medially rotate the tibia as well as approximate the medial joint.

 TIP:
The last 7.5 cm of the strip must be applied directly to the anchor strip and must **not** be applied under tension. (The tape end will peel back if tension has not been released.)

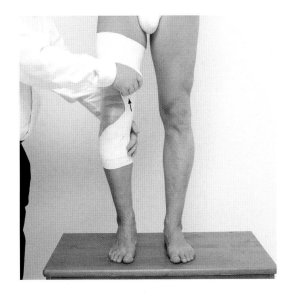

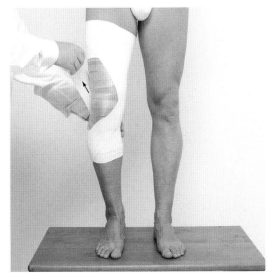

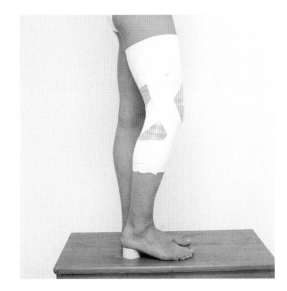

8 Place the second strip of 7.5 cm elastic adhesive bandage also starting at the posteromedial aspect of the distal anchor, this time heading anteriorly on the medial side. Pull proximately with strong tension over the medial joint line to the proximal anchor anteriorly, releasing the tension only when adhering the end of the strip.

 NOTE:
These two strips form an X directly on the medial joint line over the site of the medial collateral ligament.

9a Begin the lateral X with a strip of 7.5 cm elastic adhesive bandage from the posteromedial aspect, winding behind the tibia (reinforcing internal rotation of the tibia) with some tension upwards on the lateral aspect of the knee above the patella to the proximal anchor anteriorly.

 NOTE:
These last two strips form an X directly on the lateral joint line, with less tension. The ends interlock with the medial X over the anchors, reinforcing stability.

9b Place the next strip of 7.5 cm elastic adhesive bandage from the anterolateral aspect of the distal anchor, pulling proximally with some tension over the lateral joint line, to the proximal anchor.

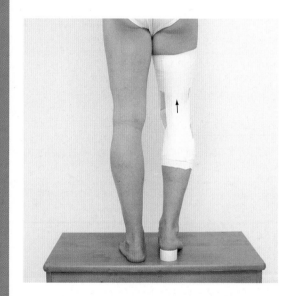

10 With the knee still flexed, apply a vertical strip of 7.5 cm elastic adhesive bandage from the centre of the posterior of the distal anchor to the centre of the proximal anchor to prevent hyperextension.

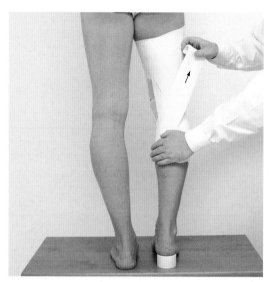

11 Apply an X of 7.5 cm elastic adhesive bandage (fully stretched) on the posterior knee.

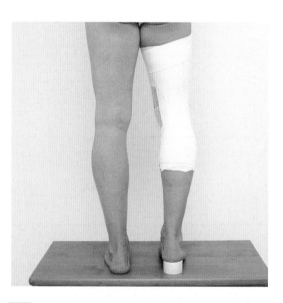

12 Re-anchor the tape proximally and distally.

NOTE:
This completed butterfly must be tight enough to limit the last 10–15° of knee extension.

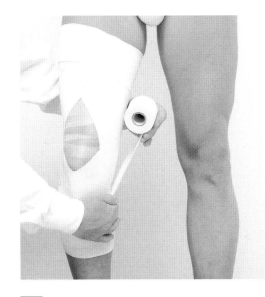

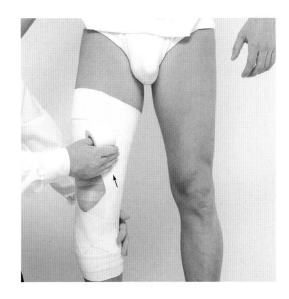

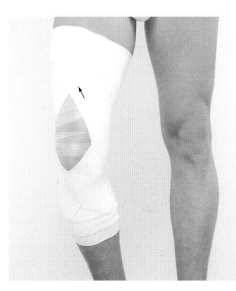

13 Apply an oblique vertical strip of 5 cm non-elastic tape from the posteromedial aspect of the distal anchor to the anteromedial aspect of the proximal anchor.

 TIP:
Fold the edges of the tape back on themselves to reinforce its strength, making the portion crossing the ligament virtually untearable.

 TIP:
When applying this strip, hold the distal end firmly against the distal anchor while pressing the knee into extreme varus and pull up with maximal force.

 NOTE:
The athlete will need to hold on to the taper's shoulder or a nearby wall for stability at this stage.

 NOTE:
The knee must remain relaxed while the athlete's weight is borne mainly on the uninjured leg.

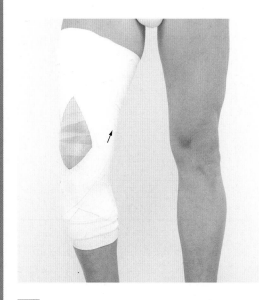

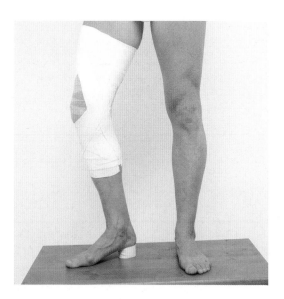

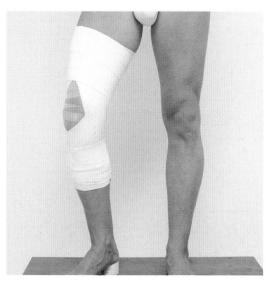

14 Apply a second vertical strip of non-elastic tape, this time from the anterior aspect of the distal anchor to the posteromedial aspect of the proximal anchor using the same principles as outlined in step 12.

15 Repeat the non-elastic tape X, overlapping slightly anteriorly to the first tape.

16 Using light tension, re-anchor the tape job with two circumferential strips of 10 cm elastic adhesive bandage over the midthigh and midcalf anchors.

NOTE:
The X formed by these two strips must lie on the medial line over the site of the MCL.

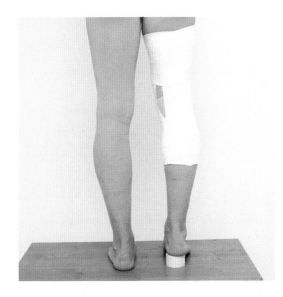

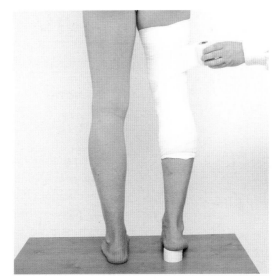

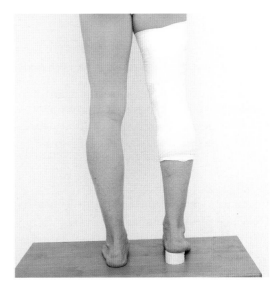

17 Cover the end of the elastic tape with two short strips of non-elastic tape to keep the elastic tape securely in place.

18 Test the degree of restriction.
  a. Extension must be limited by 10°.
  b. There must be no medial laxity.
  c. There must be no pain on medial stress testing, external rotation of the tibia under the femur or extension.

19 Wrap the entire tape job with an elastic wrap prior to allowing the athlete to resume activity. This gives the tape the time and heat necessary to set.

20 Tape the elastic wrap in place with non-elastic tape.

NOTES:

- For acute sprains, leave elastic wrap on for at least the first 48 hours.

- For back-to-sport taping, leave the elastic wrap on for 15 minutes and then remove for full activity.

ANATOMICAL AREA: KNEE AND THIGH

INJURY: KNEE SPRAIN MEDIAL COLLATERAL LIGAMENT

T ERMINOLOGY

- medial collateral ligament sprain: 1st–3rd degree of severity (see Sprains chart, p. 36)
- internal collateral ligament sprain: 1st–3rd degree of severity
- pulled knee

E TIOLOGY

- excessive inward pressure forcing the knee medially into valgus (inwardly bent 'knock-kneed' position). Example: a football player tackled at the knees from the left side may sustain a medial sprain of the left knee and potentially a lateral sprain of the right knee
- sudden impact forcing body laterally on a fixed foot
- often associated with other injured structures (medial meniscus, medial collateral ligament and anterior cruciate ligament: 'the unhappy triad')

S YMPTOMS

- local pain and tenderness on the medial side (inside) of the knee
- swelling, possible bruising
- active movement testing: medial pain on end-range extension
- resistance testing (neutral position): no pain on moderate resistance
- stress testing:
    a. 1st- and 2nd-degree sprain: medial pain with or without instability when tested at 30° knee flexion
    b. 3rd degree of severity: complete ligament rupture 'opens up' at 30°, can be less pain than with 2nd degree
    c. **instability at 0°** extension is indicative of a severe injury with posterior capsule involvement

T REATMENT

Early

- R.I.C.E.S.
- Taping: **MCL sprain, p. 136** (plus elastic wrap for first 48 hours)
- therapeutic modalities

Later

- continued therapy including:

 NOTE:
Surgery may be indicated for 3rd-degree sprain.

    a. therapeutic modalities

    b. transverse friction massage

    c. mobilizations if stiff following immobilization

    d. flexibility exercises for quadriceps, hamstrings and gastrocnemii

- strengthening exercises (isometric at first) for quadriceps and hamstrings
- gradual reintegration programme with pain-free taped support: **for MCL sprain,** see p. 136
- total rehabilitation programme for range of motion, flexibility, strength and proprioception
- bracing may be recommended for return to activity or for continued athletic performance if chronically unstable

S EQUELAE
- medial (valgus) laxity
- chronic instability
- weakness of quadriceps
- degeneration of medial meniscus
- osteoarthritic changes

R.I.C.E.S.: Rest, Ice, Compress, Elevate, Support.

TAPING FOR LATERAL COLLATERAL LIGAMENT SPRAINS OF THE KNEE

Purpose

- supports the lateral collateral ligament (LCL) by tightening the lateral aspect of the joint line
- prevents the last 15° of knee extension and restricts end-range flexion slightly
- allows functional flexion and extension of the knee

Indications for use

- lateral collateral ligament sprains: 1st and 2nd degree
- post immobilization of 3rd-degree LCL sprains
- can be combined effectively with taping techniques MCL or for multiple knee ligament injuries

MATERIALS

Razor
Skin toughener spray/adhesive spray
Underwrap
Lubricant
Heel and lace pads
10 cm (4 in) elastic adhesive bandage
7.5 cm (3 in) elastic adhesive bandage
5 cm (2 in) non-elastic white bandage
15.2 cm (6 in) elastic wrap

NOTES:

To determine degree of injury, be certain that a competent sports medicine specialist examines the athlete.

  a. lateral stability should be tested at 30° knee flexion and at 0°.

  b. if the knee is also unstable medially at 0° extension, a serious injury is indicated.

  c. X-rays should be taken.

- Be certain to check both medial and lateral sides of both knees for damage resulting from lateral impact.
- Watch for peroneal nerve damage, weakness of eversion (outward pushing) of foot and decreased sensation – lateral side of injured leg.
- Keep tabs on any necessary medical follow-up.
- Ensure that anchor tightness does not compromise circulation.

For additional details regarding an injury example see T.E.S.T.S. chart, p. 149.

Positioning

Standing upright. Place a roll of tape under the heel of the foot of the injured knee, so that the knee is slightly flexed. The foot is turned inwards to medially rotate the tibia under the femur (releasing the tension from the MCL); 80% of the body weight should be supported by the uninjured side.

Procedure

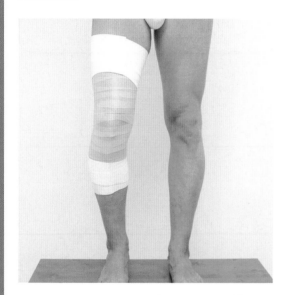

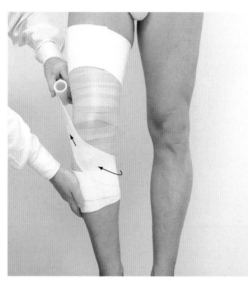

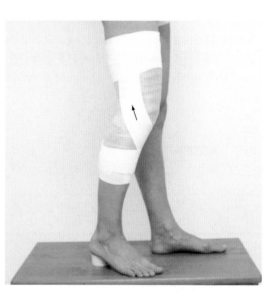

1 Make sure the area to be taped is clean and relatively hair free. Check skin for cuts, blisters or areas of irritation before spraying with skin toughener or spray adhesive.

2 Apply skin toughener/adhesive spray, skin lubricant pads, underwrap and anchors as illustrated in previous technique. **For more detail, see steps 2–5 of MCL Taping**.

TIP:
Apply lubricant and padding on both hamstring tendons to protect tender skin from irritations, blisters and tape cuts.

3 Begin the lateral 7.5 cm elastic adhesive bandage X with a strip starting anteriorly on the distal anchor, pulling up strongly around the tibia, and lateral to the patella, finishing on the proximal anchor posteriorly.

TIP:
For stability, have the athlete place a hand on the taper's shoulder or use a nearby wall or other stable structure for support during the taping procedure, particularly during application of the lateral support arrows.

NOTE:
Be sure to maintain the knee in as much valgus as possible in order to keep the lateral aspect shortened.

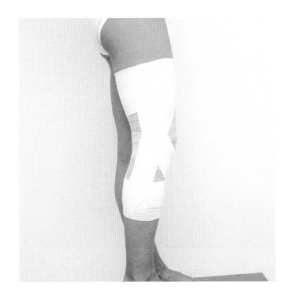

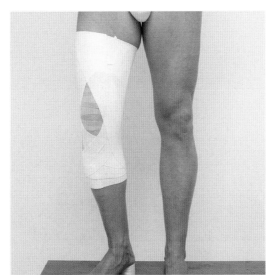

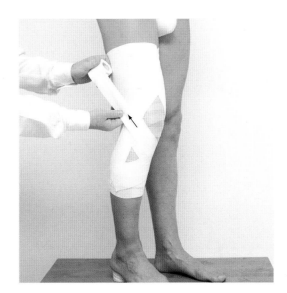

4 Complete the lateral X with a strip from the posterolateral distal anchor, pulling up strongly to the anterolateral proximal anchor, with the X over the lateral joint line.

5 Repeat anchor X on the medial aspect without causing internal rotation of the tibia or varus (outward) stress on the knee.

 NOTE:
Avoid compressing the patella when taping.

6 Use a vertical strip of 5 cm non-elastic tape with the edges folded in for extra strength, to reinforce the lateral ligament. Start anteriorly on the inferior anchor and pull up strongly on the lateral side, keeping the knee in maximum varus, and adhere the tape securely to the proximal anchor posteriorly.

7

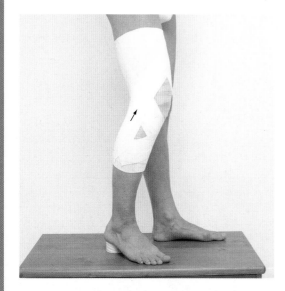

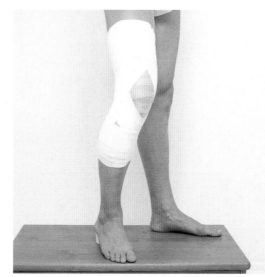

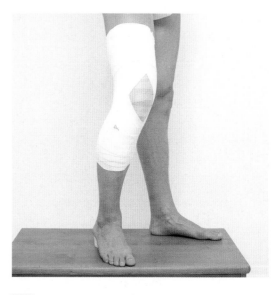

7 Complete this laterally reinforcing X with a second vertical strip starting posteriorly on the distal anchor, and crossing the previous strip at the joint line. Maintain maximal varus while adhering the end to the proximal anchor anteriorly.

NOTE:
It is important to place these crosses over the lateral joint line well behind the patella.

8 Apply the second white tape X slightly posterior to the first, with the X at the joint line.

NOTE:
- For sprains: leave elastic wrap on for at least the first 48 hours.
- For back-to-sport taping, leave elastic wrap on for at least 15 minutes and remove for full activity.

9 Remember to anchor the tape job.

10 Before applying elastic wrap, test for degree of restriction:
  a. extension must be restricted by 10°
  b. there must be no lateral laxity and
  c. there must be no pain on lateral stress testing (bending outwards) or extension.

11 **Continue with steps 16, 18 and 19 in the previous (MCL) taping, pp. 142-143.**

ANATOMICAL AREA: KNEE AND THIGH

INJURY: KNEE SPRAIN: LATERAL COLLATERAL LIGAMENT

T ERMINOLOGY
- lateral collateral ligament sprain
- external collateral ligament sprain
- fibular collateral ligament sprain
- torsion injury
- **see sprains chart, p. 36, for description of 1st to 3rd degree of severity**

E TIOLOGY
- excessive outward pressure forcing the knee laterally into varus (outwardly bent or 'bow-legged' position)
- sudden impact forcing body medially on fixed lower leg
- direct blow to side of knee
- isolated tears are uncommon

S YMPTOMS
- pain, tenderness on lateral side (outside) of the knee
- swelling, possible bruising
- active movement testing: lateral pain on end-range extension
- passive movement testing: lateral pain on end-range extension
- resistance testing (neutral position): no pain on moderate resistance
- stress testing at 0° and 30° knee flexion
  a. 1st- and 2nd-degree sprains: pain with or without instability
  b. 3rd degree of severity: complete ligament rupture ('opens up'); can be less pain than with 2nd-degree sprain. See notes re degree of injury testing (p. 36)
  c. instability at 0° extension is indicative of a severe injury with posterior capsule involvement

NOTE:
Surgery may be indicated for 3rd-degree sprain.

T REATMENT
Early
- R.I.C.E.S.
- therapeutic modalities
- taping for **LCL sprain taping (p. 145)** (plus elastic wrap for first 48 hours)

Later
- continued therapy including:
  a. therapeutic modalities
  b. transverse friction massage
  c. mobilizations if stiff after immobilization
- flexibility exercises for quadriceps, hamstrings and gastrocnemius
- strengthening of quadriceps, hamstrings and gastrocnemius
- strengthening of quadriceps (isometric at first)
- gradual reintegration programme with pain-free taped support: **LCL sprain taping, p. 145**
- total rehabilitation programme for range of motion, flexibility, strength and proprioception
- bracing may be recommended for return to activity or for continued athletics if chronically unstable

S EQUELAE
- lateral (varus) laxity
- rotational instability
- predisposition to lateral meniscal tears
- weakness of quadriceps
- inability to 'cut' when running
- possible peroneal nerve damage
- degenerative arthritic changes

R.I.C.E.S.: Rest, Ice, Compress, Elevate, Support.

TAPING FOR PATELLO-FEMORAL PAIN

Purpose

- compresses the patellar tendon, thereby changing lines of stress and thus altering the biomechanics of the patello-femoral joint
- reduces upward mobility of patella
- allows full movement at the knee joint

Indications for use

- patellar tendinitis
- patello-femoral joint syndrome
- Osgood–Schlatter's disease
- medial knee pain associated with flat feet (seek advice from podiatrist on foot orthotics)
- 'jumper's knee'

NOTES:

- Evaluate pain using a visual analogue score (VAS) prior to taping, by having the athlete perform a half-squat. Re-evaluate this movement throughout the taping procedure, monitoring any change in pain. Use only the taping strips which alleviate the pain.

- Avoid compressing the patella against the femur, as this may aggravate pain.

- There should be no pain during activity. If the athlete cannot function pain free, a patella strap may be indicated (jumper's knee strap).

- The semi-elastic adhesive tape used in this procedure is minimally elastic and maximally adherent. Should it not be available, use non-elastic adhesive tape instead (do not use elastic adhesive bandage).

MATERIALS

Razor
Quick-drying adhesive spray
2.5 cm (1 in) semi-elastic tape (preferable) or non-elastic tape (semi-elastic tape has a minimal amount of elasticity and is not a conventional elastic adhesive tape)

For additional details regarding an injury see T.E.S.T.S. chart, p. 154.

Positioning

Relaxed, supported long sitting position or supine, with the knee aligned in a neutral position and supported on a roll or cushion.

Procedure

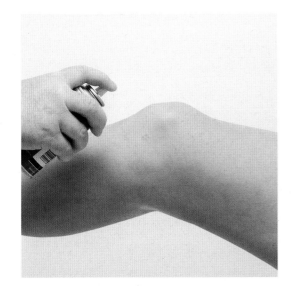

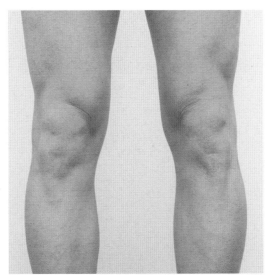

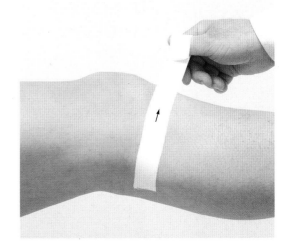

1 Make sure the area to be taped is clean and relatively hair free; shave if necessary

2 Check skin for cuts, blisters or areas of irritation before spraying with skin toughener or spray adhesive.

3 Perform the test position: a half-squat.

NOTE:
Assess the intensity of pain with a VAS, and the angle of the knee at pain onset.

4 Starting posteriorly on the lateral side, apply a horizontal strip of 2.5 cm semi-elastic adhesive tape. Using moderate firm pressure, this strip should compress the patellar tendon just above the tibial tubercle.

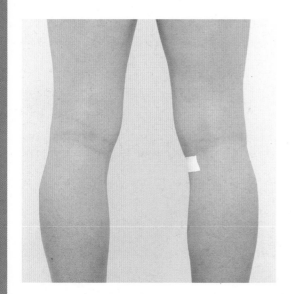

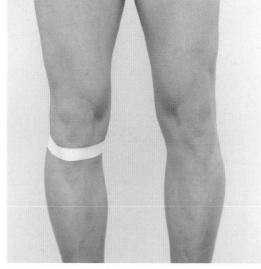

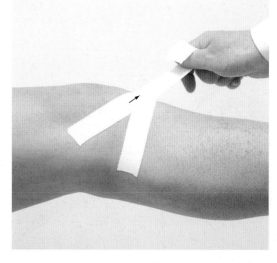

NOTE:
- Do not encircle the leg completely
- Make sure that the tape ends adhere well to the skin.

5   Re-evaluate the level of pain.

6   Apply a diagonal strip of tape from the upper lateral aspect of the knee beside the patella, pulling distally across the patellar tendon and ending medially.

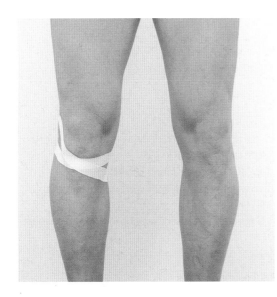

7   Re-evaluate the level of pain.

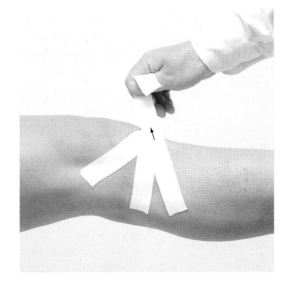

8   Apply a diagonal strip of tape from the lower lateral aspect of the knee beside the patella, pulling proximally across the patellar tendon and ending medially.

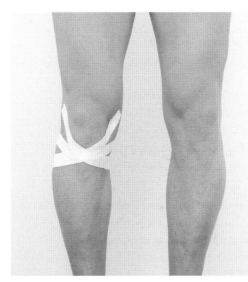

9   Re-evaluate the level of pain.
- **a.** 40° of full weight-bearing flexion should be possible.
- **b.** If pain is not eliminated with this taping, try a patellar tendon strap (jumper's knee strap).

NOTE:
Active therapy should precede returning to activity.

7

ANATOMICAL AREA: KNEE AND THIGH

CONDITION: PATELLO-FEMORAL JOINT SYNDROME

T ERMINOLOGY
- patellar malalignment syndrome
- retro-patellar inflammation
- pre-chondromalacia

E TIOLOGY
- quadriceps weakness
- poor tracking of patella
- subluxing or dislocating patella
- poor biomechanics of adjacent joints
- posttraumatic blow to knee
- secondary to patellar tendinitis
- jumping as in plyometric training
- common in basketball and volleyball

S YMPTOMS
- peripatellar pain may be experienced in various locations:
  a. diffuse around the patella
  b. at the inferior tip of the patella
  c. anterior or posterior to the patellar tendon
  d. at the tibial tubercle (insertion of the tendon)
- pain is often felt following sitting or resting
- active movement testing: may have pain on extension; pain when climbing or particularly when descending stairs
- passive movement testing: muscle tightness or imbalance involving quadriceps, hamstrings and tensor fascia lata (TFL)
- resistance testing (neutral position): weakness of quadriceps (specifically vastus medialis obliquus –VMO) with or without pain
- stress testing: patello-femoral grinding test causes pain

T REATMENT

Early

(if acutely inflamed)
- ice
- therapeutic modalities
- lateral retinacular stretching
- taping: **for Patellar Tendon, see p. 150**

Later
- continued therapy including:
  a. therapeutic modalities to control pain
  b. quadriceps re-education: particularly vastus medialis obliquus (VMO) utilizing muscle stimulation or biofeedback
  c. flexibility exercises, hamstring and tensor fascia lata (TFL)
- gradually progressive negative weight training with corrected biomechanics (proper patellar tracking) and taping
- orthotics may help if faulty alignment is caused by poor foot biomechanics

S EQUELAE
- chronic pain of quadriceps
- weakness of quadriceps and tensor fascia lata (TFL)
- inflexibility
- inability to participate in sports
- chondromalacia

Patello-femoral joint syndrome

TAPING FOR QUADRICEPS (THIGH) CONTUSION OR STRAIN

Purpose

- applies localized specific compression to the bruised or torn tissue
- prevents subsequent swelling, bleeding or muscle fibre tearing in the area
- allows full function and flexibility

Indications for use

- quadriceps contusion
- quadriceps strain
- for hamstring strains tape is applied to posterior thigh

NOTES:

- The exact site of the contusion or strain must be localized.
- Underwrap is not recommended, as it significantly lessens the effectiveness of the tape technique.
- The pressure of tape strips must be localized to the injured area and not too tight circumferentially. If constricted, hamstring and calf muscles may cramp; also, the athlete may feel that the leg is weak, stiff or heavy.
- Any massage is strictly contraindicated in the early stages due to the high risk of further internal bleeding and the potential development of myositis ossificans.

MATERIALS

Razor
Skin toughener spray/adhesive spray
10 cm (4 in) elastic adhesive tape
7.5 cm (3 in) elastic adhesive tape
3.8 cm (1½ in) non-elastic white tape
15.2 cm (6 in) elastic wrap

For additional details regarding an injury example see T.E.S.T.S. chart, p. 161.

Positioning

Lying on a bench with the knee flexed over the edge and the heel resting on the ground or the floor.

Procedure

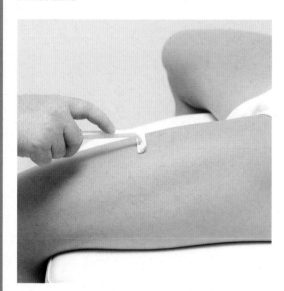

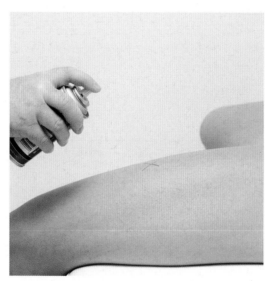

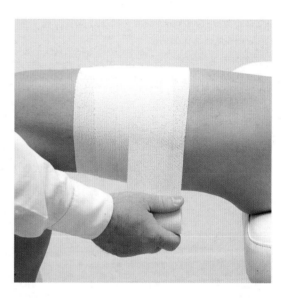

1 Make sure the area to be taped is clean and relatively hair free; shave if necessary. Check skin for cuts, blisters or areas of irritation before spraying with skin toughener or spray adhesive.

2 Localize and mark the exact site of the contusion or muscle strain.

3 Spray quick-drying adhesive circumferentially to the thigh and let dry completely.

4 Beginning 7.5 cm below the lower aspect of the injury, wrap 10 cm elastic adhesive bandage around the limb using light tension. Repeat this strip, overlapping the previous one by approximately 1.5 cm (½ in) until the entire injured area is covered and surpassed by 7.5 cm.

NOTE:
This layer of tape forms a foundation for the compression strips to avoid excessive tension on the skin.

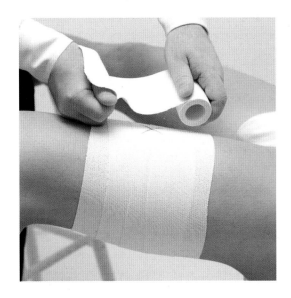

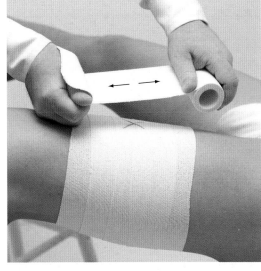

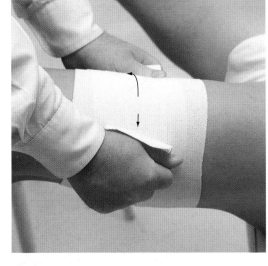

NOTE:

For large thighs or large contusions, 10 cm tape can be used for these strips if the taper has wide enough hands to maintain pressure across the entire tape width.

5 Prepare to apply the first pressure strip directly below the centre of the site of injury.

a. Fold back 12 cm (5 in) at the end of the roll of 7.5 cm elastic adhesive bandage in one hand and hold the remainder of the roll in the other.

5b Stretch the tape fully, hold it horizontally across the limb and keep it stretched laterally.

5c Apply strong pressure equally with both hands while maintaining lateral stretch until the tape reaches three-quarters of the way around the limb. Wrap the tape ends towards the back and let the roll hang down on the medial side.

NOTE:

This pressure can cause some discomfort.

TIP:

The taper can better stabilize and control counter-pressure by gripping and squeezing the athlete's knee with their own knees to gain better support during the application of the pressure strips. (Technique not illustrated.)

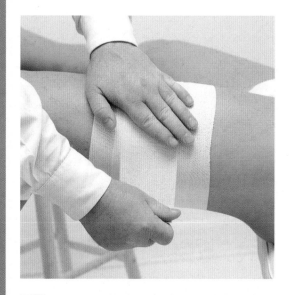

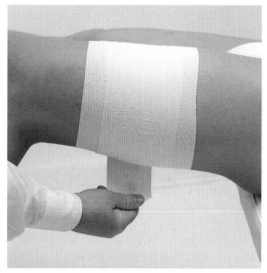

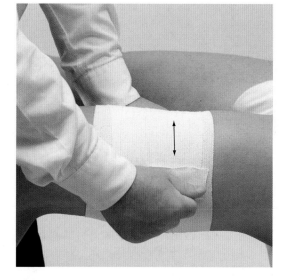

5d Be careful to keep the strip from detaching and release the tension before adhering the lateral tape end posteriorly.

5e Complete encircling the limb by overlapping the tape ends well at the back without tension.

6 Repeat the pressure strip, overlapping by half the tape width above the first strip.

7 Repeat again over the injury, always with maximal pressure anteriorly.

TIP:
Ensure the medial side does not detach while cutting the tape from the roll.

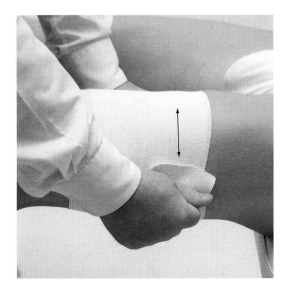

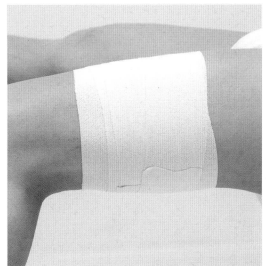

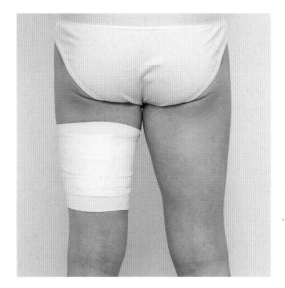

8   Continue repeating the pressure strips, overlapping by half proximally until the entire tape base is covered.

TIP:
Ensure the tape job extends at least one full tape width above and below the area of injury.

9   Finish the ends of this taping with short strips of non-elastic tape to avoid detachment of the elastic tape during activity.

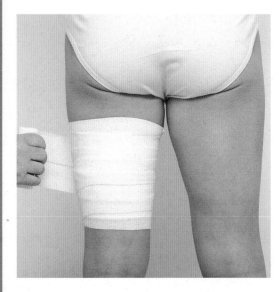

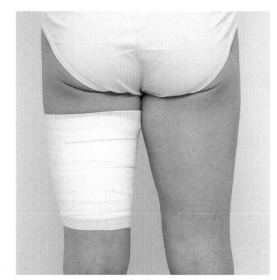

10 Wrap the entire tape job with an elastic wrap prior to activity, to give the adhesive in the tape the time and heat necessary in order to set (remove prior to activity).

11 Affix the elastic wrap with non-elastic tape.

12 Re-assess the degree of pain – isometrically, isotonically and in full dynamic motion.

ANATOMICAL AREA: KNEE AND THIGH

CONDITION: QUADRICEPS CONTUSION

T ERMINOLOGY
- contusion of one of the quadriceps muscles 1st to 3rd degree severity (**see contusion chart, p. 38**)

E TIOLOGY
- direct blow on thigh; for example, a direct blow from a tackle to the thigh in rugby or football)

S YMPTOMS
- pain, tenderness over site of injury
- swelling and haematoma if not treated immediately
- active movement testing: pain on active contraction of quadriceps
- passive movement testing:
  a. pain on knee flexion
  b. worse with hip extension
- resistance testing (neutral position): pain and/or weakness of quadriceps
- palpable localized deformity possible

T REATMENT
Early
- ice
- taping: **Compression, see p. 49**
- early flexibility exercises enhanced by active contraction of hamstrings only; no overpressure

- therapeutic modalities
- gentle activity with taped compression

Later
- continued therapy including:
  a. therapeutic modalities
  b. strengthening exercises: pain free
  c. flexibility exercises
- gradual return to full pain-free activity with taped support; see **Compression taping, p. 49**
- dynamic proprioceptive programme

S EQUELAE
- haematoma
- myositis ossificans if massaged early
- complete rupture of muscle if used too early
- weakness
- scarring and inflexibility
- predisposition to recurrent strains

7

ANATOMICAL AREA: KNEE AND THIGH

TAPING FOR ADDUCTOR (GROIN) STRAIN

Purpose

- applies localized support and compression over the injured muscles
- allows full flexion and extension
- applies local pressure while permitting full flexibility
- can also be adapted to restrict abduction

Indications for use

- acute adductor (groin) strain
- chronic adductor (groin) strain
- adductor tendinitis

NOTES:

- The exact site of injury must be localized.
- Be certain that groin injuries of the muscle attachments to the pubic bone are properly evaluated; if in doubt, **refer**.
- If necessary, X-ray to rule out avulsion or stress fractures (scans may be necessary in the early stages of a stress fracture as they may not show, initially, on X-ray) or osteitis pubis which refers pain to the adductor region.
- The skin near the groin is extremely tender and prone to irritation: careful preparation of this area is essential (a full explanation of the technique should be given to the patient prior to taping and consent sought due to the intimate nature of the groin region).
- Once taped, the usual pretraining/event stretches should be carried out with the utmost care. Proper warm-up and flexibility will reduce the risk of re-injury or an exacerbation of the current injury.

MATERIALS

Razor
Skin toughener spray/adhesive spray
10 cm (4 in) elastic adhesive bandage
7.5 cm (3 in) elastic adhesive bandage
3.8 cm (1½ in) non-elastic tape
15.2 cm (6 in) elastic wrap

For additional details regarding an injury example see T.E.S.T.S. charts, p. 166.

Adductor (groin) strain

Positioning

Standing with the knee slightly flexed, the heel on a roll of tape and the foot turned inwards (this decreases the stretch of the groin muscles). Re-check the position frequently during the course of the taping.

Procedure

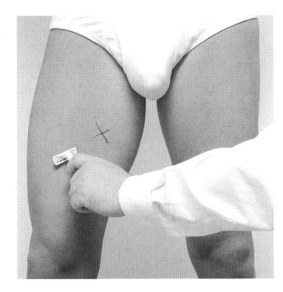

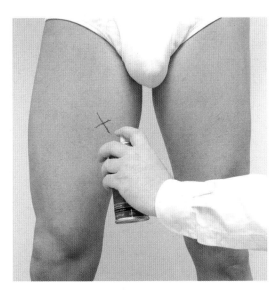

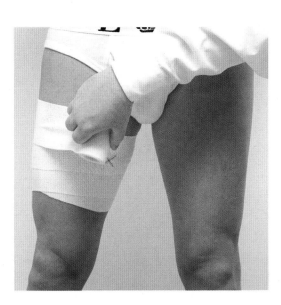

1. Make sure the area to be taped is clean and relatively hair free; shave if necessary (in cases of upper thigh and groin injury, you may want to ask the patient to do this). Check skin for cuts, blisters or areas of irritation before spraying with skin toughener or spray adhesive.

2. Localize and mark the exact site of the injury.

3. Spray skin toughener or quick-drying adhesive circumferentially to the thigh and let dry completely (care must be taken when spraying close to sensitive body areas).

4. Apply one layer of 4 cm elastic adhesive bandage with light tension around the limb.

5. Continue additional foundation strips overlapping by 2 cm until the tape covers an area of at least 7.5 cm above and below the injury site.

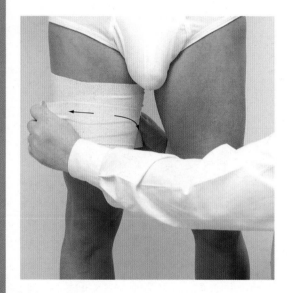

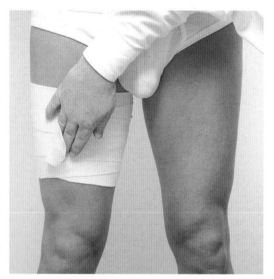

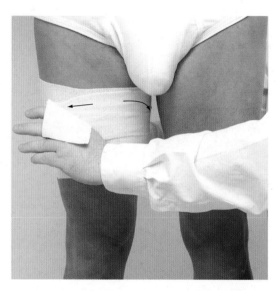

6 Apply the first pressure strip slightly below the site of the injury.
a. First stretch the tape fully and apply it with strong pressure equally with both hands. Release the pressure only when the tape strip reaches three-quarters of the way around the limb.

6b Apply the remainder of the strip ends, encircling the limb with little or no tension, being careful not to allow these to peel back and consequently lose the localized pressure.

7 Apply subsequent strips of tape proximally, overlapping by one half the width of the tape above this first strip, as in the previous technique.

NOTE:
The finished tape job should have no creases or folds.

Adductor (groin) strain

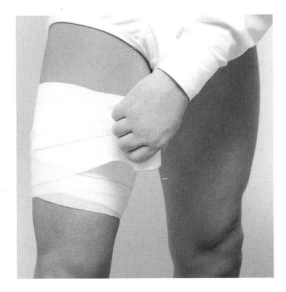

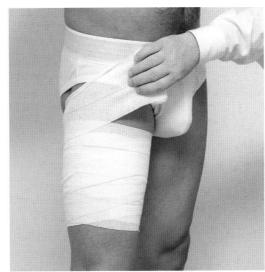

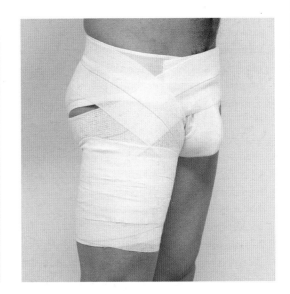

8 Cover the ends of this taping job with short strips of non-elastic tape as in the previous technique.

9 Wrap the entire tape job with an elastic wrap prior to activity, to give the adhesive in the tape the time and heat necessary in order to set, in the following fashion (hip spica technique).
a. Wrap the tensor in a modified figure of eight medially around the upper thigh.

9b Then around the hip and waist.

 TIP:
Maintain correct positioning in slight internal rotation.

10 Affix the end of the wrap with non-elastic tape.

11 Test the degree of pain reduction – isometrically, isotonically and in full dynamic motion.

 NOTE.
This 'spica' elastic wrap can be reinforced with a second wrap pulled tightly enough to assist adduction and resist abduction.

ANATOMICAL AREA: KNEE AND THIGH

INJURY: ADDUCTOR STRAIN

T ERMINOLOGY
- strain of one of the adductor muscle or tendons, severity 1st to 3rd degree
- 'pulled' groin muscle

E TIOLOGY
- explosive contraction of adductor muscles
- excessive stretch of adductor muscles
- more susceptible when muscles are not warmed up
- overuse due to unaccustomed repetitive action
- common in goal tending, soccer, hockey, football and some track and field sports

S YMPTOMS
- slight to severe pain varying with degree and location of injury
- pain may be diffuse or localized and may reach as high as pubic bone
- haematoma not always present
- active movement testing:
  a. some pain on hip adduction
  b. pain also possible on active abduction due to muscle stretch
- passive movement testing: pain on hip adduction
- resistance testing (neutral position: pain and/or weakness on hip adduction)

T REATMENT
Early
- R.I.C.E.S.
- taping: for **adductor strain taping, see p. 162**
- therapeutic modalities
Later
- continued therapy including:
  a. transverse friction massage
  b. progressive, graduated exercises to regain strength (isometric and non-weight bearing at first)
- gradual reintegration to activities programme with pain-free taped support

S EQUELAE
- persistent pain
- weakness
- scarring and inflexibility
- chronic reinjury
- imbalance may lead to pelvic and lumbar spine compensatory problems
- bone spurs may develop
- ossification of haematoma possible

R.I.C.E.S.: Rest, Ice, Compress, Elevate, Support.

The **gleno-humeral** (shoulder) joint is one of the most mobile of all the joints in the body. It is this mobility that predisposes the shoulder joint to injury, both acute and chronic, and heightens the joint's dependency on muscular and capsular support. By contrast, the **acromio-clavicular** (AC) joint is less mobile and depends solely on ligaments for support.

At the elbow, the **humero-ulnar** joint (the true elbow joint) is a hinge joint similar to the knee. It sustains similar injuries, requiring the application of taping principles presented in the knee/thigh section.

The main purpose and value of taping an elbow is the prevention of full extension of the joint, with or without lateral reinforcement. Because the associated **radio-ulnar** (forearm) joint allows a great degree of pronation and supination (rotation), the overall effectiveness of taping for lateral ligaments is compromised.

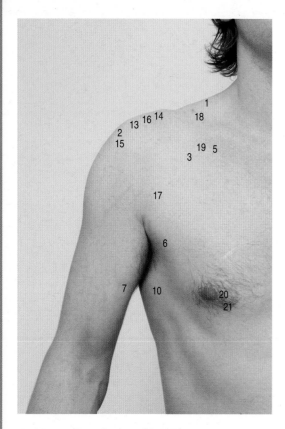

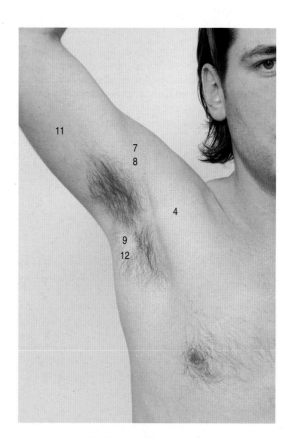

MUSCLES

1. Trapezius
2. Deltoid
3. Anterior margin of deltoid
4. Pectoralis major
5. Upper margin pectoralis major
6. Lower margin pectoralis major
7. Biceps short head
8. Coracobrachialis
9. Teres major
10. Serratus anterior
11. Triceps

TENDONS

12. Latissimus dorsi

BONES

13. Acromion of scapula
14. Acromial end of clavicles
15. Greater tuberosity of humerus

JOINTS

16. Acromioclavicular

HOLLOWS

17. Deltopectoral groove
18. Supraclavicular fossa
19. Infraclavicular fossa

MISCELLANEOUS

20. Areola
21. Nipple

Right shoulder from the front.
The arm is slightly abducted
- The nipple in the male (21) normally lies at the level of fourth intercostal space.
- The deltopectoral groove containing the cephalic vein is formed by the adjacent borders of deltoid (2) and pectoralis major (5).
- The lower border of pectoralis major (6) forms the anterior fold.

The right axilla or armpit is the hollow below the shoulder. Its anterior wall is made up mainly of the fibres of pectoralis major (4) with pectoralis minor behind. The posterior wall consists of teres major (9) with the tendon of latissimus dorsi (12) immediately in front. Close to pectoralis major a bundle of muscle made up of the short head of biceps (7) and coracobrachialis (8) runs down the arm with the cords of the brachial plexus surrounding the axillary artery immediately behind. The axilla is also a very important site for lymph glands draining lymphatics from the arm and, most importantly, the breast.

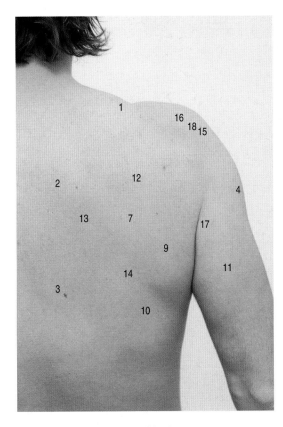

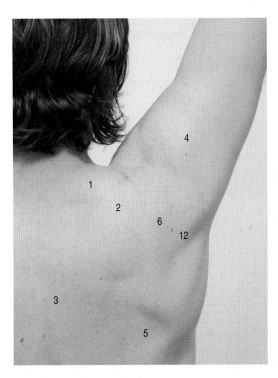

MUSCLES

1. Trapezius – upper fibres
2. Trapezius – middle fibres
3. Trapezius – lower fibres
4. Deltoid
5. Rhomboid major
6. Supraspinatus
7. Infraspinatus
8. Teres minor
9. Teres major
10. Latissimus dorsi
11. Triceps

BONES

12. Spine of scapula
13. Vertebral border of scapula
14. Inferior angle of scapula
15. Acromion of scapula
16. Acromial end of clavicle

NERVES

17. Axillary nerves posterior to humerus

JOINTS

18. Acromioclavicular

Right shoulder, from behind.
The arm is slightly abducted and the inferior angle of the scapula (14) has been made to project backwards by attempting to flex the shoulder joint against resistance.

- The inferior angle of the scapula (14) usually lies at the level of the seventh intercostal space. It is overlapped by the upper margin of the latissimus dorsi (10).
- The axillary nerve (17) runs transversely under cover of the deltoid (4) behind the shaft of the humerus at a level 5–6 cm below the acromion (15).
- Latissimus dorsi (10) and teres major (9) form the lower boundary of the posterior wall of the axilla.

Right shoulder, arm elevated.
While maintaining good postural control of the trunk, the right arm has been abducted through some 180°. The left scapula remains in a normal resting position but with firm muscle control, the glenoid pointing laterally. The right scapula has been rotated through some 70–75° under the activity of trapezius with the remaining arm movement occurring at the shoulder joint. Activity is obvious in deltoid (4), the major abductor at the shoulder joint, and no doubt in supraspinatus (6), though this muscle is masked by trapezius (2).

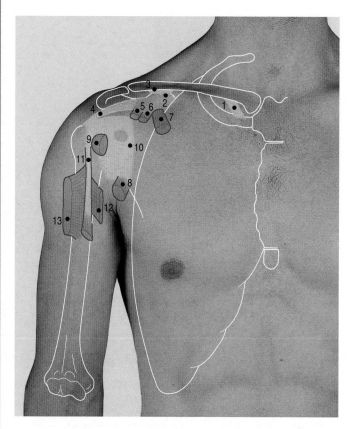

Shoulder joint: anterior aspect.
1 Costoclavicular ligament. 2 Conoid ligament. 3 Trapezoid ligament. 4 Coracohumeral ligament. 5 Short head of biceps. 6 Coracobrachialis. 7 Pectoralis minor. 8 Long head of biceps. 9 Subscapularis. 10 Anterior capsule of shoulder joint with opening of subscapular bursa. 11 Long head of biceps. 12 Latissimus dorsi. 13 Pectoralis major.

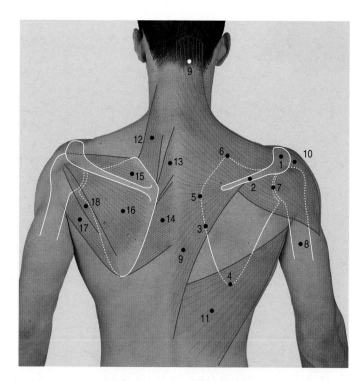

Posterior aspect of the shoulder and upper arm: bones and muscles of the shoulder girdle. Right, superficial muscles; left, deep muscles. 1 Acromion. 2 Spine of scapula. 3 Medial border of scapula. 4 Inferior angle of scapula. 5 Medial angle of scapula. 6 Superior angle of scapula. 7 Glenoid fossa. 8 Humerus. 9 Trapezius. 10 Deltoid. 11 Latissimus dorsi. 12 Levator scapulae. 13 Rhomboideus minor. 14 Rhomboideus major. 15 Supraspinatus. 16 Infraspinatus. 17 Teres major. 18 Teres minor.

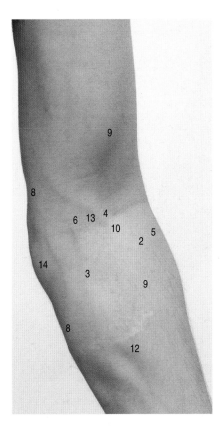

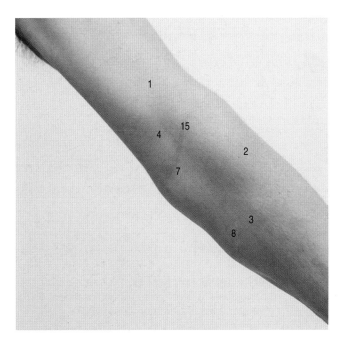

Forearm from the front.

a. Left elbow from the front. There is an M-shaped pattern of superficial veins. Cephalic (9) and basilic (8) veins are joined by a median cubital vein into which drain two small median forearm veins. The order of the structures in the cubital fossa from lateral to medial is biceps tendon (4), brachial artery (13) and median nerve (6).

MUSCLES
1. Biceps
2. Brachio Radialis
3. Pronator Teres
4. Biceps
5. Flexor carpi Radialis

NERVES
6. Median

FASCIA
7. Bicipital Aponeurosis

VEINS
8. Basilic
9. Cephalic Vein
10. Median Cephalic Vein
11. Median Basilic Vein
12. Median Forearm Vein

ARTERIES
13. Brachial

BONES
14. Medial Epicondyle of Humerus
15. Lateral Epicondyle of Humerus

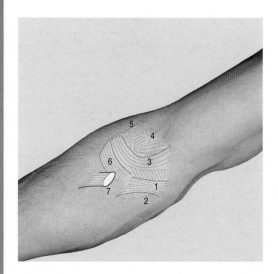

Elbow joint: anterior aspect. 1 Anterior band of medial ligament. 2 Oblique band of medial ligament. 3, 4 Anterior capsule. 5 Lateral ligament. 6 Annular ligament. 7 Tendon of biceps.

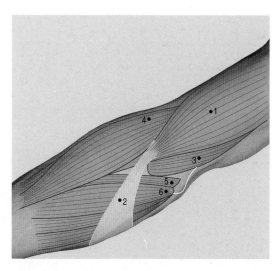

Cubital fossa: soft tissues. 1 Biceps. 2 Bicipital aponeurosis. 3 Brachialis. 4 Brachioradialis. 5 Pronator teres. 6 Common flexor origin.

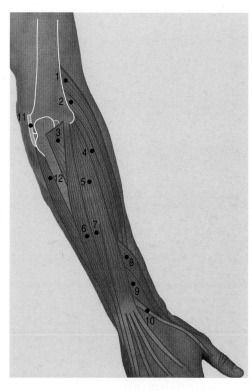

Posterior aspect of the elbow and forearm: superficial muscles. 1 Brachioradialis. 2 Extensor carpi radialis longus. 3 Anconeus. 4 Extensor carpi radialis brevis. 5 Extensor digitorum. 6 Extensor carpi ulnaris. 7 Extensor digiti minimi. 8 Abductor pollicis longus. 9 Extensor pollicis brevis. 10 Extensor pollicis longus. 11 Ulnar nerve. 12 Flexor carpi ulnaris.

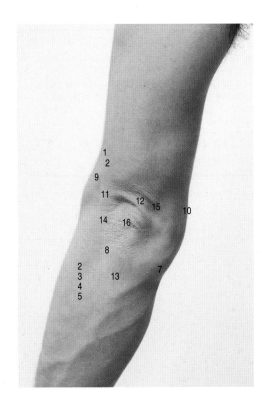

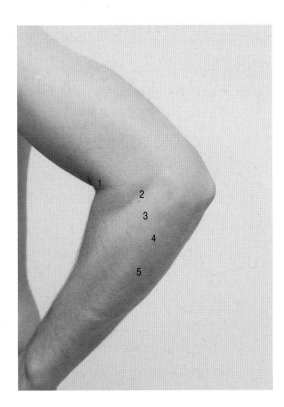

The back of the forearm

The superficial extensor muscles take a common origin from the lateral epicondyle and the supracondylar ridge. Brachioradialis (1), the muscle coming from higher up the ridge, has been described with the anterior muscles in view of its role as a flexor muscle. Extensor carpi radialis longus (2) also comes from the supracondylar ridge below brachioradialis and below that, the extensor carpi radialis brevis (3) which arises from the epicondyle. These muscles can be identified quite easily running down the radial side of the back of the forearm.

MUSCLES

1. Brachioradialis
2. Extensor carpi radialis longus
3. Extensor carpi radialis brevis
4. Extensor digitorum
5. Extensor carpi ulnaris
6. Triceps
7. Flexor carpi ulnaris
8. Anconeus

BONES

9. Lateral epicondyle of humerus
10. Medial epicondyle of humerus
11. Capitulum of humerus
12. Olecranon of ulna
13. Posterior border of ulna
14. Head of radius

NERVES

15. Ulna

BURSA

16. Margin of the olecranon bursa

Left elbow from behind

With the elbow fully extended, the extensor muscles form a bulge in the lateral side. In the adjacent hollow can be felt the head of the radius (14) and the capitulum of the humerus (11) which indicates the line of the radio-humeral part of the elbow joint. The lateral and medial epicondyles (9, 10) of the humerus are palpable on either side. Wrinkled skin lies at the back of the prominent olecranon of the ulna (12). In this arm the margin of the olecranon bursa (16) is outlined. A very important structure in this region is the ulnar nerve (15) which is palpable as it lies in contact with the humerus behind the medial epicondyle (10). The posterior border of the ulna (13) is subcutaneous throughout its whole length.

- With the elbow extended, the medial and lateral epicondyles and the olecranon are on the same level but with flexion of the elbow, the olecranon moves to a lower level.
- The subcutaneous position of the ulnar nerve behind the medial epicondyle makes it easily palpable. Here it can be easily injured, causing paraesthesia (tingling) in the distribution of the ulnar side of the hand. This area is commonly referred to as the 'funny bone'.

8

Shoulder and Elbow

TAPING FOR ACROMIOCLAVICULAR (AC) SPRAIN: SHOULDER SEPARATION

Purpose

- compresses and stabilizes the acromioclavicular (AC) joint
- keeps the distal end of the clavicle down while allowing almost full gleno-humeral function
- elastic support assists abduction

Indications for use:

- acute AC sprain
- sub-acute shoulder separation
- chronic shoulder separation
- chronic step deformity accompanied by pain at the AC joint

MATERIALS

Rectangular piece of felt or very dense foam approximately 5 × 3.6 cm (2 × 1½ in) and 1 cm (½ in) thick to cover AC joint
Square of gauze, thin felt or folded underwrap approximately 3.6 × 3.6 cm (2 in sq) to cover nipple
Razor
Skin toughener spray/adhesive spray
3.8 cm (1½ in) non-elastic tape
7.5 cm (3 in) elastic adhesive bandage
5 cm (2 in) elastic adhesive bandage

TIP:
Ensure that step deformity is corrected/reduced by proper positioning.

NOTES:

- Acutely injured athletes should not return to competition without proper investigation (high risk of advancing severity of the injury).
- Ensure correct diagnosis by following up with a sports medicine specialist.
- Be certain that a radiological evaluation is done, particularly if any deformity is present.
- This taping can be used for a female athlete by applying the chest anchors below the breasts and the anterior end of the vertical anchor angled more towards the midline.
- Monitor limb sensation, strength of pulse and venous return prior to, during and after taping to ensure that there is no neurovascular compromise.
- Tender skin at the axilla (armpit) needs special attention and protection.

For additional details regarding an injury example see T.E.S.T.S. chart, p. 181.

Positioning
Sitting comfortably with the elbow and forearm well supported across the lap with a solid cushion.

Procedure

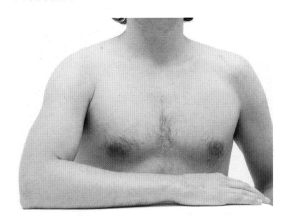

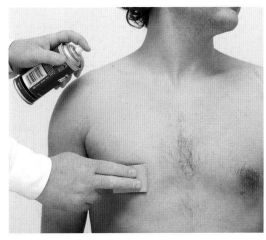

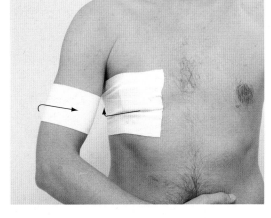

1   Make sure the area to be taped is clean and relatively hair free; shave if necessary.

2   Check skin for cuts, blisters or areas of irritation before spraying with skin toughener or spray adhesive

NOTE:
Sensation, pulse, temperature and colour must be checked before starting to tape.

NOTE:
Alternatively, fixation tape can be used in conjunction with adhesive spray and fixed halfway round the mid-humerus from front to back, instead of encircling the upper arm.

3   Spray the area well with tape adherent to maximize adhesiveness, thus stabilizing anchors.

TIP:
Turn athlete's face away and protect nipple when spraying.

4   Wrap an anchor with light tension around mid-humerus with 7.5 cm (3 in) elastic adhesive bandage.

TIP:
Ensure that the last 7.5 cm (3 in) ends of the anchors are applied without tension and pressed firmly to avoid 'peeling back' of the tape.

5   Apply two anchors of 7.5 cm elastic adhesive bandage horizontally to the chest with light pressure, from anterior to posterior at the level of the 5th rib (covering the nipple with gauze, underwrap or felt, especially in men).

Acromioclavicular (AC) sprain: Shoulder separation

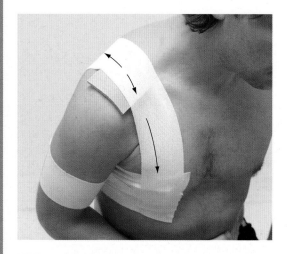

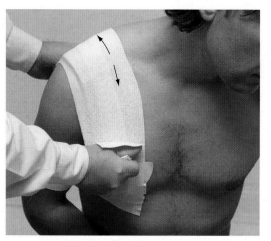

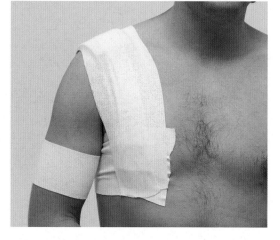

6 Cut a piece of felt or dense foam padding large enough to cover the prominence of the AC joint (approx. 3.5 × 5 cm and at least 1 cm thick).

7 Using 7.5 cm elastic adhesive bandage and moderate tension, apply rectangle directly on the upper end of the AC joint (outer tip of the clavicle and adjacent acromion).

8 Apply a compression strip of tape directly downwards over the distal end of the clavicle. Extend the elastic tape horizontally as much as possible and apply through the padding with strong pressure downwards while maintaining the horizontal tension. Release the tension only when the ends of the strip reach the chest anchor anteriorly and posteriorly (front and back).

9 Repeat this strip, moving laterally to cover one half of the first strip.

NOTE:
Recheck sensation, pulse, temperature, colour.

TIP:
Be sure the athlete is still sitting well positioned with the forearm supported.

TIP:
Ensure that the last 7.5 cm of tape is completely without tension when being affixed.

Acromioclavicular (AC) sprain: Shoulder separation

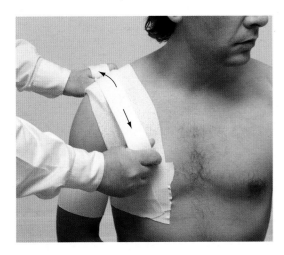

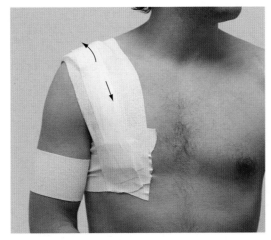

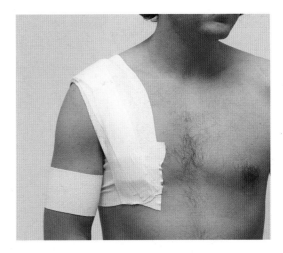

10 Reinforce stability by applying a strip of 3.8 cm non-elastic tape.
a. Maintain strong horizontal tension while applying strong pressure downwards on the superior (upper) aspect of the AC padding.

b. Ensure that these strips cross the anchor completely.

11 Apply a second downwards strip of non-elastic tape more laterally.

TIP:
Do not release tension until the anchors are reached.

NOTE:
These strips further stabilize the distal end of the clavicle and approximate the normal anatomical position of the joint.

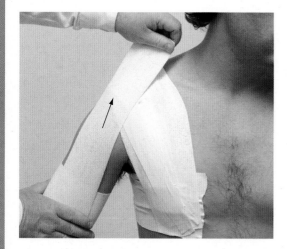

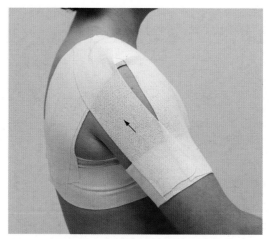

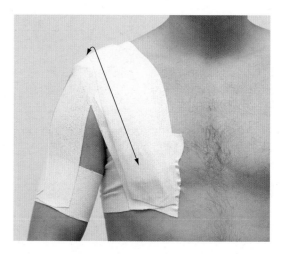

12   **a.** Re-anchor over the chest anchor to hold strips in place.

b. With arm at approximately 45° angle of abduction (ask the patient to put their hand on their hip), place a strip of 7.5 cm elastic adhesive bandage, starting laterally from the arm anchor, going anteriorly across the top of the padding and pulling up with firm tension to take the weight of the arm off the distal part of the joint.

13   Repeat this strip, starting posterolaterally on the arm and pulling up on the posterior aspect of the deltoid muscle.

NOTE:

When properly placed, the combination of these two strips assists abduction.

14   Anchor the top of these strips with a strip of elastic adhesive bandage.

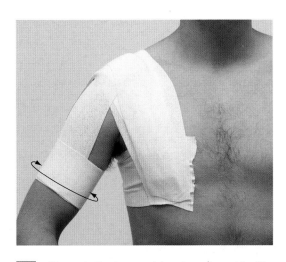

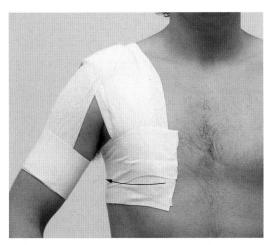

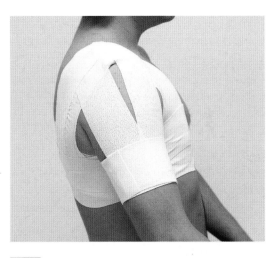

15 Reapply the humeral (arm) anchor strip (if using fixation tape go just beyond the ends of the tape front and back so skin contact is made).

16a Finish with a strip of elastic adhesive tape, applied as a horizontal anchor to the chest, to fix the lower ends of the vertical strips of tape.

 NOTE:
Re-test sensation, pulse, temperature and colour, ensuring that taping has not compromised circulation.

16b Lateral view of finished taping.

17 Assess the degree of pain reduction post taping – static and with unassisted arm flexion and abduction.

 TIP:
During the acute phase a sling or collar and cuff may be used to support the weight of the arm.

 NOTE:
The arm section of the tape job becomes optional as the AC responds to treatment and becomes less problematic.

ANATOMICAL AREA: SHOULDER AND ELBOW

INJURY: SHOULDER SPRAIN ACROMIOCLAVICULAR (AC) SEPARATION

T ERMINOLOGY
- sprain of acromioclavicular joint: 1st to 3rd degree of severity

E TIOLOGY
- direct impact to the point of the shoulder
- a fall, landing on the tip of the shoulder
- a severe fall on the outstretched arm
- common in hockey, rugby, football, horse riding and martial arts

S YMPTOMS
- pain and tenderness over the top of the AC joint
- local swelling and bruising
- active movement testing: pain on all movements, particularly on flexion and horizontal adduction
- resistance testing: pain on all movements
- passive movement testing: pain on horizontal adduction
- stress testing: varying degrees of pain and step deformity between the clavicle and the acromion in 2nd and 3rd degrees of sprain severity

T REATMENT
Early
- R.I.C.E.S.
- taped support: a sling can offer additional support during first 48 hours
- therapeutic modalities
- 2nd- and 3rd-degree sprains should have at least 3 weeks of inactivity and support before dynamic treatment is started

NOTE:
Severe 3rd-degree shoulder sprains may require surgery.

Later
- continued therapy including:
  a. therapeutic modalities
  b. range of motion and flexibility exercises
  c. strengthening: isometric at first
  d. carefully guided progressive functional strengthening as tolerated
- gradual return to pain-free sports activity with taped support
- a felt doughnut over the joint can further protect it from impact in contact sports

NOTES:
Premature return to activity risks further injury, escalating a 2nd-degree sprain to a 3rd-degree sprain (complete rupture).

No muscles directly cross the AC joint, therefore muscle strengthening does not specifically reinforce it.

S EQUELAE
- instability
- chronic pain
- associated strain of deltoid or trapezius muscles can cause residual weakness
- arthritic changes: osteophyte formations
- 'clicking'

R.I.C.E.S.: Rest, Ice, Compress, Elevate, Support

ANATOMICAL AREA: SHOULDER AND ELBOW

TAPING FOR ELBOW HYPEREXTENSION SPRAIN

Purpose

- supports the elbow laterally
- limits the last 30° of extension and end-range pronation of the forearm
- allows full flexion and almost full supination

Indications for use

- acute, sub-acute or chronic hyperextension sprains of the elbow
- posterior impingement syndrome
- medial sprains of the elbow, supported by reinforcing the medial **X** strips
- lateral sprains of the elbow, supported by reinforcing the lateral **X** strips
- combination ligament sprains
- chronic instability following fracture, dislocation of the elbow

MATERIALS

Razor
Skin toughener spray/adhesive spray
Underwrap
5 cm (2 in) elastic adhesive bandage
7.5 cm (3 in) elastic adhesive bandage
3.8 cm (1½ in) non-elastic adhesive tape
7.5 cm (3 in) elastic wrap bandage

NOTES:

- Ensure a proper diagnosis by a sports medicine specialist.
- X-rays should be taken to rule out possibility of fracture.
- Pain or laxity on lateral stress testing with the elbow at 15° flexion will indicate the need for added medial or lateral support.
- Easily irritated structures include the biceps tendon, soft skin in elbow crease and the ulnar nerve or 'funny bone', found posteromedially in the groove.
- If forearm anchor is too tight, circulation of the forearm will be constricted.

For additional details regarding an injury example see T.E.S.T.S. chart, p. 187.

Positioning

Sitting, with the elbow held in 40° flexion. The forearm should be in a neutral position between pronation and supination with the hand in a functional position.

Procedure

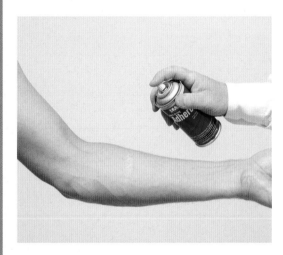

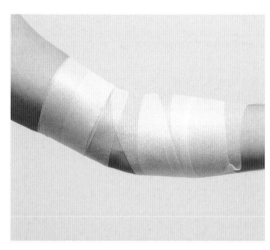

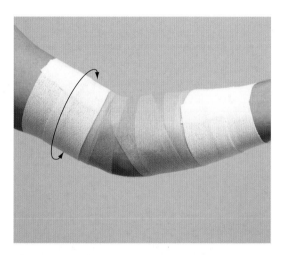

1 Make sure the area to be taped is clean and relatively hair free; shave if necessary.

2 Check skin for cuts, blisters or areas of irritation before spraying with skin toughener or spray adhesive.

 NOTE:
Sensation, pulse, temperature and colour of hand must be checked prior to taping.

3 Apply underwrap from the proximal (upper) one-third of the forearm to the distal (lower) one-third of the humerus.

 NOTE:
Padding and lubricant may be applied on the anterior aspect of the elbow to protect the biceps tendon and the soft skin when returning to sports with significant repetitive elbow motion.

4 Apply two circumferential anchors of 5 cm elastic adhesive bandage with minimal tension to the mid-humerus half-covering the underwrap and half-covering the skin directly.

5 Repeat two similar anchors mid to lower forearm.

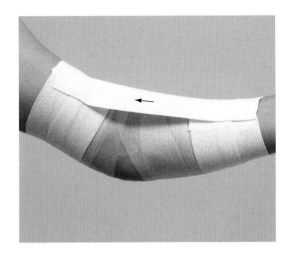

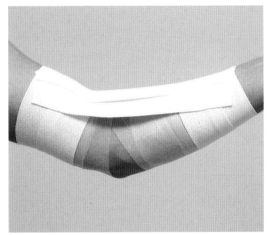

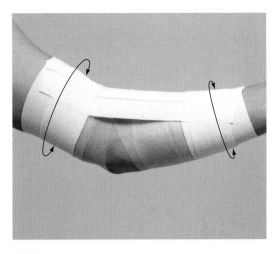

6 To form a check-rein, place the elbow in 45° of flexion and apply a vertical strip of 5 cm elastic adhesive bandage from the lower anchor with tension to the upper anchor, directly over the anterior aspect of the elbow joint.

7 Repeat this strip, overlapped by half the tape width more laterally.

8 Anchor these strips at both ends.

TIP:
Remember to keep the hand in a functional position.

TIP:
Be certain to apply these strips with enough tension to block the last 30° of extension when the elbow is fully stretched.

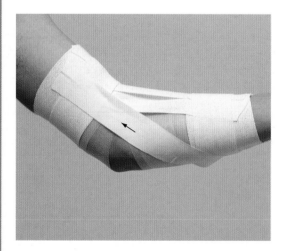

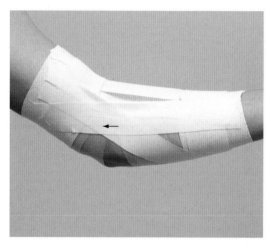

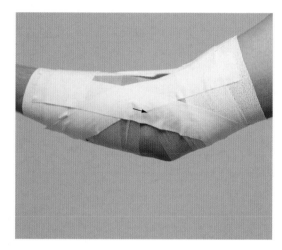

9 For medial stability, hold the elbow bent at 35° of flexion and apply a vertical strip of 3.8 cm non-elastic tape from the distal anchor to the upper anchor with strong tension.

10 Apply a second strip to form an X across the medial joint line of the elbow, also with strong tension.

NOTE:
For medial sprains ensure a varus (inwardly bent) position and apply a second white tape X on the medial side with great tension.

11 Repeat the white tape X on the lateral aspect to cross at the lateral joint line.

NOTE:
For lateral sprains ensure a more valgus (outwardly bent) position and apply a second white X on the lateral side with great tension.

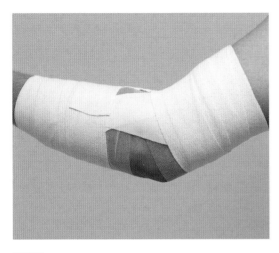

12a Apply two anchors distally and proximally using 7.5 cm elastic adhesive bandage.

NOTE:

In closing up, a space is left at the anterior elbow, to avoid undue irritation to the sensitive underlying structures.

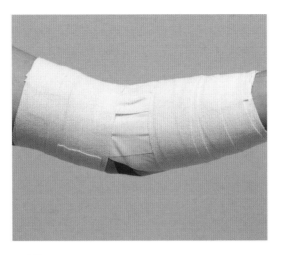

12b Anterior view of finishing taping.

NOTE:

Hand sensation, pulse, temperature and colour must be reassessed to ensure that taping has not compromised circulation.

13 Test the degree of restriction:
   a. extension should be limited by 30° or more
   b. there should be no pain on passive extension or lateral stress testing.

TIP:

Wrap the tape job with a 7.5 cm (3 in) tensor bandage for 10 minutes to ensure good adherence.

ANATOMICAL AREA: SHOULDER AND ELBOW

INJURY: ELBOW SPRAIN: HYPEREXTENSION

T ERMINOLOGY
- sprain of medial or lateral collateral ligaments
- tearing of anterior joint capsule

E TIOLOGY
- fall on outstretched hand
- forced hyperextension of the elbow (anterior capsule with/without medial and/or lateral ligament sprain)
- forced valgus (inward) stress causes damage to the medial collateral ligament (more vulnerable and more common)
- forced varus (outward) stress causes damage to the medial collateral ligament
- chronic medial sprains are common in pitchers and javelin throwers

S YMPTOMS
- pain on anterior capsule – medial and/or lateral joint line – implies localized injury site
- swelling
- active movement testing: pain on end-range extension
- resistance testing (neutral position):
  a. no significant pain on moderate resistance
  b. pain on flexion if biceps simultaneously injured
- stress testing: varying degrees of pain and laxity on stress testing (done at 15° flexion). Amount of laxity indicates degree of injury

TREATMENT
Early
- R.I.C.E.S.
- sling
- therapeutic modalities

NOTE:

NOTE: Any suspicion of deformity requires immediate medical attention and X-rays.

Later
- continued therapy including:
  a. therapeutic modalities
  b. taping for limited activity
  c. gentle traction and mobilization
- progressive resistance rehabilitation programme for humero-ulnar as well as radio-ulnar joints
- gradual return to activities with taped support as above

SEQUELAE
- chronic instability
- ulnar nerve paraesthesia
- adhesions causing reduced range of motion
- arthritic changes
- calcification of ligaments

R.I.C.E.S.: Rest, Ice, Compress, Elevate, Support.

The **wrist** is a flexible osseo-ligamentous complex forming a connective link between the forearm and the hand. Multidirectional mobility results from the numerous multiarticular carpal bones which, along with the radio-ulnar joints, allow the hand to be positioned functionally at any angle. Stability is derived from the complex array of ligaments often injured when falling on an outstretched hand.

The **hand**, while being the most active and intricate joint complex in the body, is the least protected. Constructed as a series of complex, delicately balanced joints, it offers manipulating ability, dexterity and precision. This highly sensitive structure, used to hold, catch and manipulate, is particularly vulnerable to trauma when subjected to repetitive stresses or impact of falls.

Providing adequate support while maintaining functional movement is the prime consideration when taping the hand and or wrist.

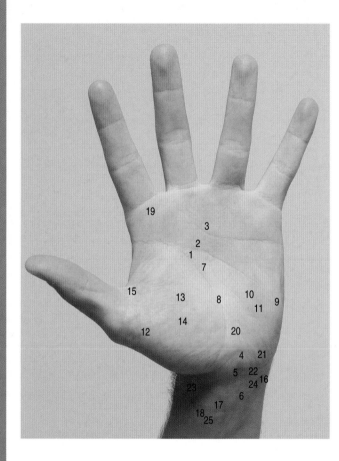

Palm of the left hand

The surface markings of various structures within the wrist and hand are indicated. Not all of them are palpable, e.g. the superficial and deep palmar arches (7, 8), but their relative positions are important.

- The curved lines proximal to the base of the fingers indicate the ends of the head of the metacarpophalangeal joints.
- The creases on the fingers indicate the level of the interphalangeal joints.
- The middle crease at the wrist indicates the level of the wrist joint.
- The radial artery at the wrist (23) is the most common site for feeling the pulse. The vessel is on the radial side of the tendon of flexor carpi radialis (18) and can be compressed against the lower end of the radius.
- The median nerve at the wrist (25) lies on the ulnar side of the tendon of flexor carpi radialis (18).
- The ulnar nerve and artery at the wrist (22, 23) are on the radial side of the tendon of flexor carpi ulnaris (16) and the pisiform bone (21). The artery is on the radial side of the nerve and its pulsation can be felt, though less easily than that of the radial artery (23).
- Abductor pollicis brevis (12) and flexor pollicis brevis (13), together with the underlying opponens pollicis, are the muscles which form the thenar eminence – the 'bulge' at the base of the thumb. Abductor digiti minimi (9) and flexor digiti minimi brevis (10), together with the underlying opponens digiti minimi, form the muscles of the hypothenar eminence, the less prominent bulge on the ulnar side of the palm where palmaris brevis (11) lies subcutaneously.

CREASES

1. Longitudinal
2. Proximal transverse
3. Distal transverse
4. Distal wrist
5. Middle wrist
6. Proximal wrist

ARCHES

7. Superficial palmar
8. Deep palmar

MUSCLES

9. Abductor digiti minimi
10. Flexor digiti minimi
11. Palmaris brevis

12. Abductor pollicis
13. Flexor pollicis brevis
14. Thenar eminence
15. Adductor pollicis

TENDONS

16. Flexor carpi ulnaris
17. Palmaris longus brevis
18. Flexor carpi radialis

BREVIS BONES

19. Head of metacarpal
20. Hook of hamate
21. Pisiform

ARTERIES

22. Ulnar
23. Radial

NERVES

24. Ulnar
25. Median

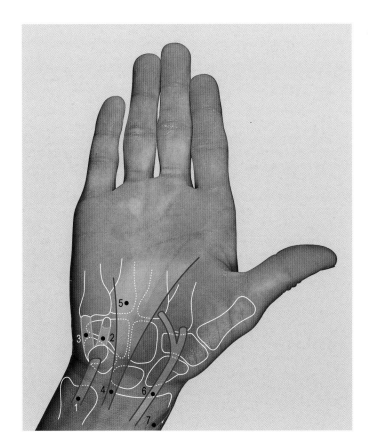

Anterior aspect of the wrist and hand: superficial tendons. 1 Flexor carpi ulnaris. 2 Pisohamate ligament. 3 Pisometacarpal ligament. 4 Palmaris longus. 5 Palmar aponeurosis. 6 Flexor carpi radialis. 7 Radial artery.

SURFACE ANATOMY

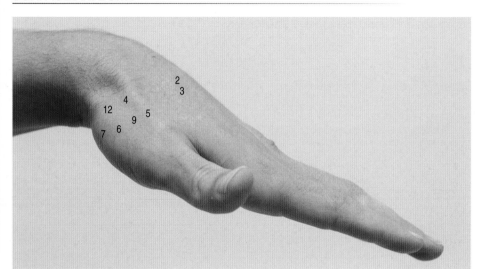

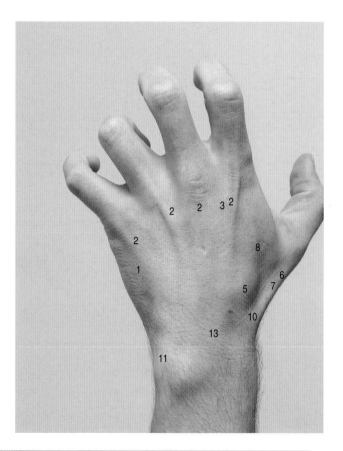

Dorsum of the left hand

The fingers are extended at the metacarpophalangeal joints, causing the extensor tendons of the fingers (1, 2 and 3) to stand out, and partially flexed at the interphalangeal joints. The thumb is extended at the carpometacarpal joint and partially flexed at the metacarpophalangeal and interphalangeal joints. The lines proximal to the bases of the fingers indicate the ends of the heads of the metacarpophalangeal joints. The anatomical snuffbox (9) is the hollow between the tendons of abductor pollicis longus (7) and extensor pollicis brevis (6) laterally and extensor pollicis longus medially (5).

TENDONS

1. Extensor digiti minimi
2. Extensor digitorum
3. Extensor indicis
4. Extensor carpi radialis longus
5. Extensor pollicis longus
6. Extensor pollicis brevis
7. Abductor pollicis longus

MUSCLES

8. First dorsal interosseus

BONES

9. Anatomical snuffbox over scaphoid
10. Styloid process of radius
11. Head of ulna

VEINS

12. Cephalic

RETINACULUM

13. Extensor retinaculum

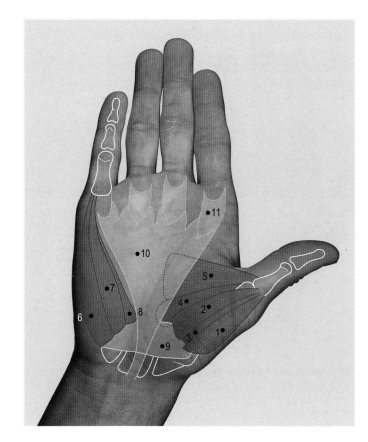

Thenar and hypothenar eminences. 1 Abductor pollicis brevis. 2 Flexor pollicis brevis. 3 Opponens pollicis. 4 Adductor pollicis oblique head. 5 Adductor pollicis transverse head. 6 Abductor digiti minimi. 7 Flexor digiti minimi. 8 Opponens digiti minimi. 9 Flexor retinaculum. 10 Palmar aponeurosis. 11 Flexor fibrous sheaths.

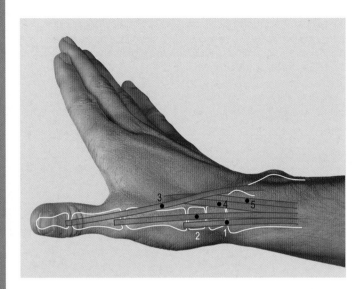

Anatomical snuffbox: tendons. 1 Abductor pollicis longus. 2 Extensor pollicis brevis. 3 Extensor pollicis longus. 4 Extensor carpi radialis longus. 5 Extensor carpi radialis brevis.

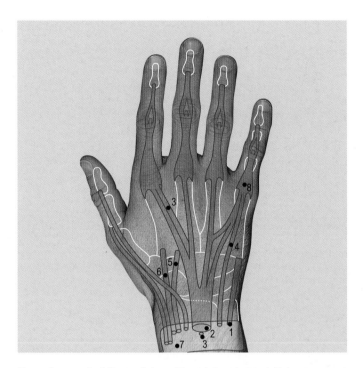

Dorsal aspect of the wrist and hand: tendons. 1 Extensor carpi ulnaris. 2 Extensor digitorum. 3 Extensor indicis. 4 Extensor digiti minimi. 5 Extensor carpi radialis brevis. 6 Extensor carpi radialis longus. 7 Extensor retinaculum. 8 Extensor digital expansion.

ANATOMICAL AREA: WRIST AND HAND

WRIST HYPEREXTENSION SPRAIN TAPING

Purpose

- reinforces the collateral ligaments of the wrist and the anterior joint structures
- restricts extension and limits the last degrees of radial and ulnar deviation
- permits functional use of the hand

Indications for use

- palmar radio-carpal ligaments sprains (hyperextension)
- for dorsal radio-carpal ligament (hyperflexion): apply the check-reins dorsally and add restraining Xs to the dorsal aspect, thus limiting end-range of flexion
- for radial collateral ligament sprain: reinforce the lateral X and add lateral palmar X to prevent ulnar deviation
- for ulnar collateral ligament sprain: reinforce the medial X and add medial palmar X to prevent radial deviation
- diffuse pain in the wrist due to repeated compression or 'jamming' the wrist
- wrist pain post immobilization

NOTES:

- Ensure that the proper diagnosis has been made to rule out fractures, particularly if the injury was caused by an outstretched hand (the scaphoid bone is the most commonly fractured).
- Clarify the mechanism of injury, whether it was hyperflexion or hyperextension that occurred.
- The use of skin toughener or quick-drying adhesive spray is essential for good adherence of taping, especially in rainy or hot conditions when hands, wrists and forearms can become quite damp.
- Wrap the circumferential strips with minimal tension, to avoid neurological or vascular compromise.
- Monitor circulatory status and sensation prior to, during and after taping.

MATERIALS

Razor
Skin toughener spray/adhesive spray
Underwrap
3.8 cm (1½ in) non-elastic tape

For additional details regarding an injury example see T.E.S.T.S. chart, p. 199.

Positioning

Sitting, with the wrist in a neutral position held in slight extension (approximately 20°).

TIP:
The elbow can be supported on a table for added stability (not shown).

Procedure

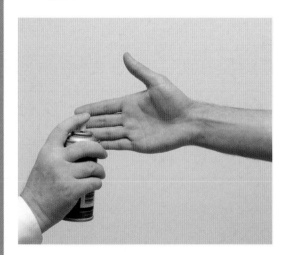
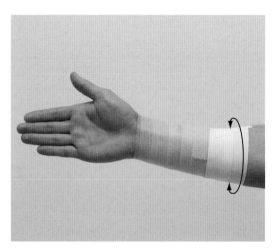
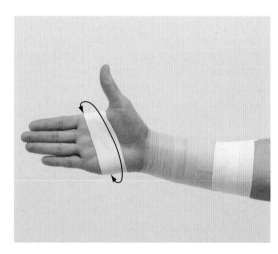

1 Make sure the area to be taped is clean and relatively hair free; shave if necessary.

2 Check skin for cuts, blisters or areas of irritation before spraying with skin toughener or spray adhesive.

3 Apply underwrap to forearm.

4 Apply two circumferential anchors of 3.8 cm non-elastic tape around the mid forearm at the musculo-tendinous junction, following the natural contours of the forearm.

5 Apply a circumferential anchor of non-elastic tape around the distal metacarpals (palm of hand).

TIP:
Ensure that these anchors do not unduly restrict the splaying of the metacarpals.

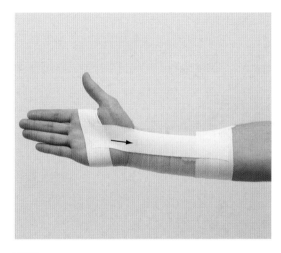

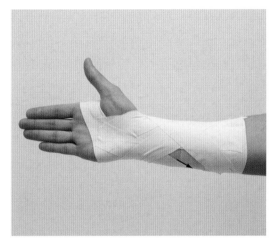

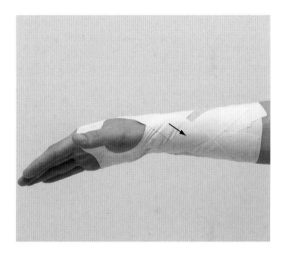

6 Hold the wrist in the neutral position and apply a check-rein from the anterior aspect of the distal anchor to the proximal, with strong tension, passing across the anterior joint line.

NOTE:
A second check-rein can be added, overlapping the first by a half for added strength and/or for wide wrists (not illustrated).

7 Start the medial X from the palmar aspect of the distal anchor to the posteromedial aspect of the proximal anchor.

8 Finish this X with a strip from the dorsal aspect of the distal anchor to the proximal anchor anteriorly with firm tension.

NOTE:
The X formed by these two strips should cross on the anteromedial joint line.

9 Begin lateral X with a strip from the dorsal aspect of the distal anchor, pulling with tension to the anterior aspect of the proximal anchor.

10 Finish this X with a strip from the palmar aspect of the distal anchor to the lateral aspect of the proximal anchor.

NOTE:
The X formed by these two strips should cross on the anterolateral joint line.

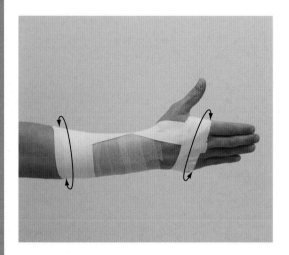

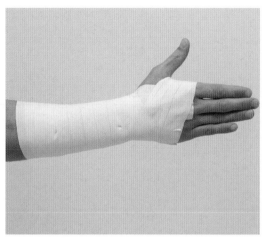

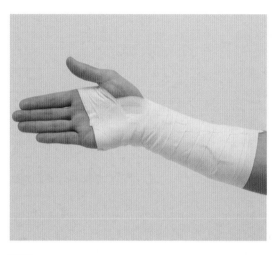

11 Re-anchor these supporting Xs both distally and proximally.

 NOTE:
For added stability, posterior Xs can be added at this time, holding the wrist in 20° or less of extension (not illustrated).

12 Close up the hand portion of the taping by overlapping the distal anchor by half the width of the next circumferential strip of non-elastic tape.

13 Continue closing up by overlapping with light circumferential strips.

14 Test the degree of restriction: extension should be limited enough to cause no pain on passive extension at the wrist.

 NOTE:
Check finger colour and sensation for signs of compromised circulation.

ANATOMICAL AREA: WRIST AND HAND

INJURY: WRIST HYPEREXTENSION SPRAIN

T ERMINOLOGY
- partial or complete tearing of anterior wrist capsule
- partial or complete tearing of radial and/or ulnar collateral ligaments

E TIOLOGY
- fall on outstretched hand
- forced hyperextension during a tackle with an opponent
- overloaded weight lifting

S YMPTOMS
- pain over anterior joint capsule and ligaments
- decreased range of motion
- swelling
- active movement testing: pain on end-range extension
- passive movement testing:
  a. pain on extension
  b. pain possible on end-range flexion resulting from compression of injured tissues
- resistance testing (neutral position): no significant pain with moderate resistance; pain possible on flexion if flexors also involved
- stress testing: varying degrees of pain and laxity

NOTE:
If wrist is unstable when testing ligaments, X-rays must be taken to rule out the possibility of fracture.

T REATMENT
Early
- R.I.C.E.S.
- initially: elastic tensor compression and sling support with careful attention to circulation for the first 48 hours
- therapeutic modalities, contrast baths

Later
- continued therapy including:
  a. therapeutic modalities
  b. flexibility exercises
  c. strengthening (isometric initially)
- total rehabilitation programme for mobility, flexibility, strengthening and dexterity
- taping for gradual return to pain-free functional activities

NOTE:
Sprains that do not respond well to treatment should be reassessed by a hand specialist. Pain and clicking on the ulnar side may imply damage to the triangular fibro-cartilage (meniscus). Persistent pain on the radial side may indicate a necrosis or missed fracture of the scaphoid.

S EQUELAE
- tenosynovitis
- weakness
- chronic sprain
- instability
- degenerative joint changes
- stubborn cases may suggest an associated meniscal tear and require some form of splinting for dynamic activity

R.I.C.E.S.: Rest, Ice, Compress, Elevate, Support.

ANATOMICAL AREA: WRIST AND HAND

THUMB SPRAIN TAPING

Purpose

- supports the collateral ligaments of the first metacarpophalangeal joint (MCPJ)
- prevents the last degrees of extension, limits abduction
- allows some flexion
- does not compromise wrist and hand function

Indications for use

- MCPJ sprain (ulnar ligament)
- carpo-metacarpal joint (CMCJ) sprain (ulnar aspect); reinforce the diagonal anchor
- 'skier's thumb', 'gamekeeper's thumb'
- post-immobilization tenderness
- after surgery of 3rd-degree repair

MATERIALS

Razor
Skin toughener spray/adhesive spray
Underwrap
3.8 cm (1½ in) non-elastic tape
2.5 cm (1 in) non-elastic tape

NOTES:

- If 3rd-degree sprain is suspected, a hand surgeon should be seen as early as possible.
- X-rays will rule out the possibility of an avulsion fracture.
- Thoroughly inspect the hand for cuts, abrasions and any other possible sources of infection.
- Watch carefully for signs of restricted circulation, particularly during the first 48 hours post injury when swelling tends to be greatest.
- Restricted circulation, apart from causing discomfort, can be particularly dangerous in below freezing weather (increased risk of frostbite).
- Hand and thumb size will dictate the width of tape required.

For additional details regarding an injury example see T.E.S.T.S. chart, p. 206.

Positioning

Sitting with the thumb and hand held in a neutral, functional position.

Procedure

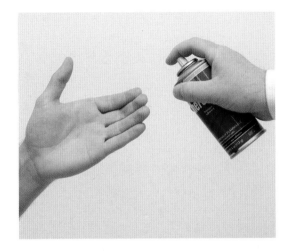

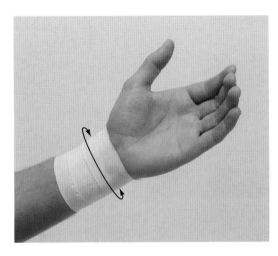

1   Make sure the area to be taped is clean and relatively hair free; shave if necessary. Check skin for cuts, blisters or areas of irritation before spraying with skin toughener or spray adhesive.

2   Apply two circumferential strips of 3.8 cm non-elastic tape around the wrist using light tension.

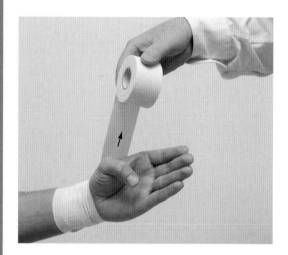

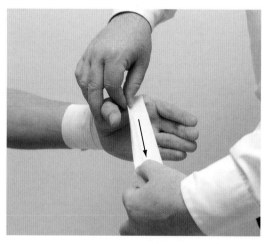

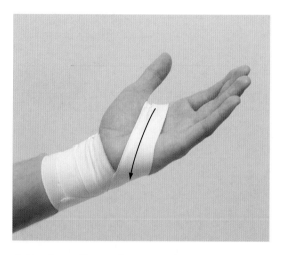

3 Apply distal anchor.
a. Using 3.8 cm non-elastic tape, start from the posterior side of the proximal anchor, wrap around the wrist, pull up and across the dorsum of the hand.

b. Cross from posterior to anterior between the thumb and index finger.
c. Pinch the tape as it passes through the web of the space to avoid irritating the soft skin at this site.

 TIP:
Be careful not to apply any pressure through the web space.

d. Continue diagonally across the palmar aspect of the hand and fix the strip medially on the proximal anchor.

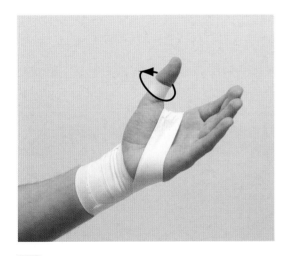

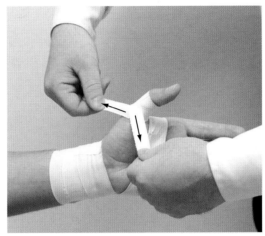

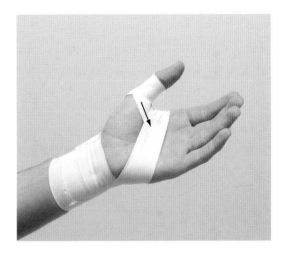

4 Apply the thumb anchor lightly, placing the strip circumferentially around the proximal phalanx, following its contours using 2.5 cm non-elastic tape (use a narrower tape if necessary).

5 Apply an incomplete figure-of-eight strip of 1.2 cm non-elastic tape by pulling gently around the thumb, crossing the strips and pulling equally with both hands medially, adducting the thumb before adhering both ends of this strip to the anchor.

6 The anterior end is applied to the palmar anchor, and the posterior end is applied to the dorsal anchor with firm pressure.

TIP:
Be careful not to apply strong pressure circumferentially around the thumb during application of tape.

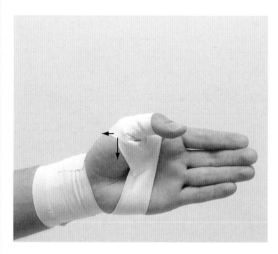

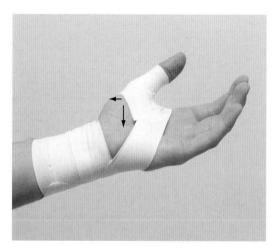

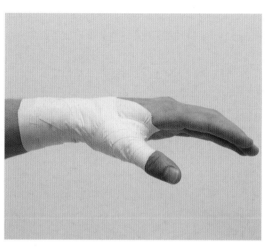

7a Apply another half figure of eight more proximally, overlapping by half the width of the tape on the thumb anchor.

7b Allow the strip ends to fan out slightly before they reach the anchor.

8 Continue repeating the half figure of eights, overlapping by half to three-quarters the width of the tape, moving proximally down the thumb.

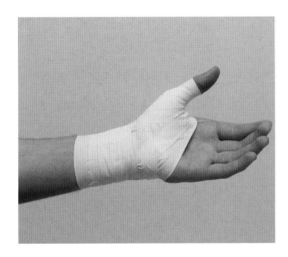

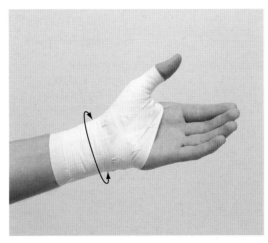

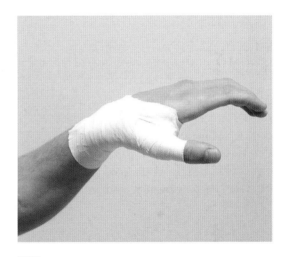

9 Re-anchor the ends of the incomplete figure of eights with another diagonal anchor.

TIP:
Be careful not to apply strong pressure through the web space.

NOTE:
A figure-of-eight check-rein can be applied between the thumb and first finger to further restrict abduction (not illustrated).

10 Apply circumferential strips of 3.8 cm non-elastic tape around the wrist, covering the diagonal anchor and any remaining tape ends.

11 Check functional position of the hand and test the degree of restriction: extension and abduction must be limited enough that there is no pain on passive movements, especially extension and abduction.

NOTE:
Check thumb colour and sensation for signs of compromised circulation.

ANATOMICAL AREA: WRIST AND HAND

INJURY: THUMB SPRAIN

T ERMINOLOGY
- partial or complete tearing of ulnar collateral ligament: the first MCPJ; degree of severity 1st–3rd
- 'game-keeper's thumb'
- 'skier's thumb'

E TIOLOGY
- forced extension and/or abduction of the MCPJ
- a fall on an outstretched hand, common in skiing

S YMPTOMS
- tenderness over medial aspect of the MCPJ
- local swelling and/or discolouration
- active movement testing: pain on end-range extension
- passive movement testing: pain on extension plus abduction
- resistance testing (neutral position): no significant pain on moderate resistance

T REATMENT
Early
- R.I.C.E.S. for first 48 hours
- therapeutic modalities; contrast baths
- range of motion (ROM) exercises
- taping: **for Thumb Sprain, see p. 200**

NOTE:
Third-degree and severe 2nd-degree sprains require spica splinting, casting or surgery with at least 3 weeks of immobilization.

Later
- continued therapy including:
  a. therapeutic modalities
  b. joint mobilizations if stiff post immobilization
  c. strengthening (isometric at first)
- gradual return to pain-free functional activities with taped support
- complete rehabilitation programme including range of motion, flexibility, strengthening and dexterity

S EQUELAE
- chronic instability with severe dysfunction
- weakness of grip
- tenosynovitis
- degenerative changes of MCPJ

R.I.C.E.S.: Rest, Ice, Compress, Elevate, Support.

ANATOMICAL AREA: WRIST AND HAND

FINGER SPRAIN TAPING

Purpose
- supports the palmar and collateral ligaments of the finger
- prevents full extension
- allows full flexion

Indications for use
- palmar ligament sprain (hyperextension) of the finger
- post-immobilization painful stiffness of the finger
- 'jammed' or 'stubbed' finger
- medial collateral ligament (MCL) sprain of the finger: reinforce medial **X**
- lateral collateral ligament (LCL) sprain of the finger: reinforce lateral **X**

NOTES:
- Never allow the athlete to continue playing (even when taped) if a serious injury is suspected.
- Ensure a correct diagnosis by a doctor or hand specialist. (Fractures and dislocations are often misdiagnosed and mistreated.)
- Localize the exact site of the injury – which aspect of which joint of which finger – and re-test for pain through range during and after the tape job is completed.
- Taping the injured finger to its neighbour ('buddy taping') further protects the injured ligaments while allowing function and movement.
- If the athlete needs to use the injured hand to handle a ball during a game, 'buddy tape' the fingers slightly apart to allow better control of the ball.

MATERIALS

Razor
Skin toughener spray
1.2 cm (½ in) Non-elastic tape

For additional details regarding an injury example see T.E.S.T.S. chart, p. 211.

Positioning

Sitting with the elbow supported on a table and the finger(s) placed in a neutral, functional position (approximately 20° flexion).

Procedure

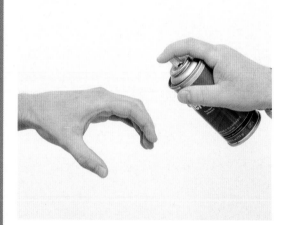

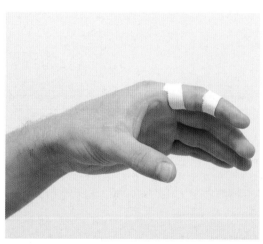

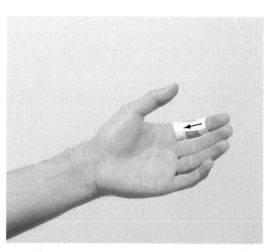

1 Make sure the area to be taped is clean and relatively hair free; shave if necessary.

2 Check skin for cuts, blisters or areas of irritation before spraying with skin toughener or spray adhesive.

TIP:
A cotton-tip applicator can be used to minimize the adherence of non-affected digits.

3 Gently apply two circumferential anchors of 1.2 cm non-elastic tape, one above and one below the injured joint.

TIP:
Be careful to avoid constriction.

4 Apply a vertical strip of 1.2 cm (½ in) white tape from the distal anchor to the proximal anchor on the centre of the volar (under) aspect of the finger, with strong tension, keeping the finger flexed about 20°.

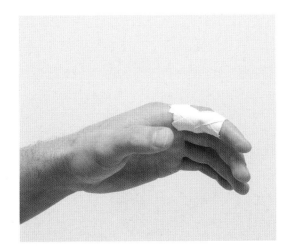

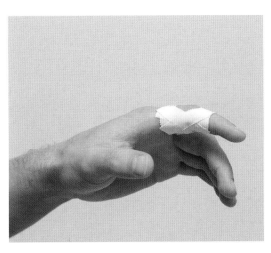

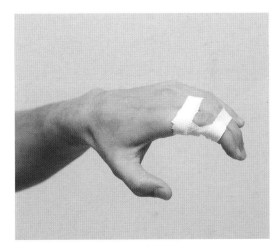

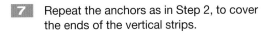

5 Apply a lateral X with two strips from the distal anchor to the proximal, with strong tension, forming the X on the lateral joint line.

6 Repeat the above on the medial aspect, with the X lying on the medial joint line.

7 Repeat the anchors as in Step 2, to cover the ends of the vertical strips.

8 Perform a simple 'buddy-taping' technique by taping the injured finger to its neighbour.

NOTE:
This step is useful for sports not needing full hand function (as in soccer, excluding goalkeeper), when the fingers can function as a unit.

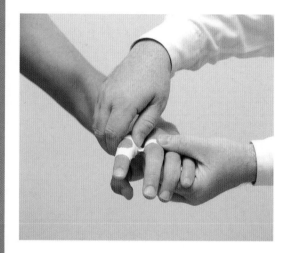

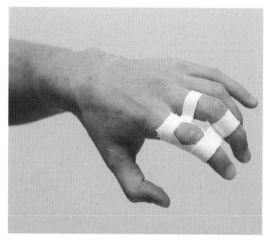

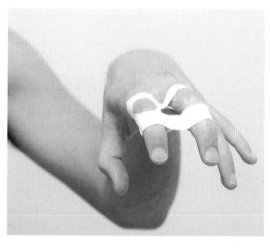

9 Alternative method: apply a webbed 'buddy-taping' by keeping the injured digit slightly abducted (spread apart) while taping it to its neighbour.

NOTE:
This technique is useful for sports requiring full functional dexterity and use of individual fingers (as in basketball or volleyball). Note that more space is left between the fingers with this option.

10 Pinch the buddy tape strip between the fingers to allow some independent movement of the injured digit.

11 Check for functional dexterity and verify adequate limits of taping.

NOTE:
Finger colour and sensation must be checked for signs of compromised circulation.

12 Test the degree of restriction: extension must be limited enough that there is no pain on stressing the injured ligament.

ANATOMICAL AREA: WRIST AND HAND

INJURY: FINGER SPRAIN

T ERMINOLOGY
- partial or complete rupture of palmar ligament (anterior capsule), medial collateral (ulnar) ligament or lateral collateral (radial) ligaments: degree of severity, 1st–3rd
- 'stoved' finger
- 'jammed' finger

E TIOLOGY
- telescoping blow: direct compressive force on the tip of the finger (i.e. jamming it against a ball as in basketball, volleyball or rugby)
- torsional stresses
- sideways stress to a finger: may catch on clothing, equipment or terrain
- hyperextension of finger
- contusion of ligaments

S YMPTOMS
- pain over site of injury
- swelling and discolouration
- local tenderness
- active movement testing: pain on end-range extension and/or flexion (pinching the injured capsule)
- passive movement testing: pain on end-range extension and/or possibly on flexion
- resistance testing (neutral position): no significant pain on moderate resistance
- stress testing:
  a. pain with or without laxity on lateral stress testing in 1st- and 2nd-degree sprains
  b. instability with 3rd-degree sprains (often with less pain)

T REATMENT

Early
- R.I.C.E.S.
- initial taping: loose **Buddy Taping, see p. 210**
- therapeutic modalities; contrast baths
- range of motion exercises

NOTE:
Third-degree and severe 2nd-degree sprains usually require splinting with at least 1 week of complete immobilization and 2 weeks of mobilization between treatments and range of motion (ROM) exercises, followed by 8 weeks of taped support.

Later
- continued therapy including:
  a. therapeutic modalities
  b. mobilizations
  c. flexibility
- strengthening exercises for all hand musculature
- taping for gradual return to pain-free functional activities
- progressive exercises for range of motion, strength and dexterity

S EQUELAE
- persistent laxity (instability)
- chronic sprain reinjury
- deformity
- stiffness
- degenerative joint changes

R.I.C.E.S.: Rest, Ice, Compress, Elevate, Support.

If you ask a patient what brings them to your clinic, or ask an athlete what stops them training or competing, they will not answer with: I think I have a problem with balance or I have too much inversion of my ankle or too much extension at my elbow. They will tell you that **pain** is the primary reason for their visit and, in the case of athletes, possibly a reduction in performance as well. Pain is quite possibly the most complex issue presented to any practitioner,[1] and among the most confounding presentations to treat.

The effects of tape and its ability to reduce pain are fairly well documented,[2-15] especially with regards to, but not limited to, the knee.[2,3,7,8,10,11,13-15] Studies have been done on other areas of the body, such as the ankle, hip, shoulder, elbow, foot and even ribs.[4-6,9,12] Some researchers are looking at the effects of tape on pain in stroke sufferers.[5,16]

In order for us to understand the reasons for pain reduction, we need to know the reasons for pain. This may at first sight seem simple, as in many cases the answer will be swelling of the tissues caused by trauma. During inflammation, pain is caused by chemical, mechanical and thermal irritants. Taping for this aspect of pain has already been adequately dealt with in the other sections of this book. However, this does not explain chronic pain or why many suffer discomfort long after the original injury has healed. For this we have to look to other areas for the answers. It would be a reasonable statement to say that other factors are multifactoral and therefore, by their very nature, complex. Two such theories have been hypothesized as possible reasons for maintenance of painful joints, represented by Panjabi and his hypothesis of a 'neutral zone'[17,18] and Dye's hypothesis on joint homeostasis.[19-21] Both are very feasible and have led to further research in these areas.

The need for pain reduction has prompted some tapers to look at other ways of obtaining maximal pain-alleviating effects by using tape. In some cases the more traditional tried and tested methods of taping may be inappropriate or contraindicated. In several cases, as the injury recovers less tape is needed to offer the same effect (limit joint range of motion and pain relief). McConnell describes a method of pain-relieving taping as 'unloading' and stated that: 'tape may be used to unload painful structures to minimize the aggravation of the symptoms so treatment can be directed at improving the patient's "envelope of function" '.[2]

There are at present three primary taping techniques used:

- athletic taping
- McConnell taping
- Kinesio Taping®.

Athletic taping is by far the most widely used technique and is primarily used for acute injuries and prevention of injuries (as well as all the reasons laid out in the introduction). It is generally applied prior to a sporting activity and removed immediately after.

McConnell (unloading) taping was devised and researched by Jenny McConnell. It was primarily designed for patellofemoral joint syndrome. It uses a highly adhesive fixation tape in combination with a non-elastic tape. It is also used on other areas such as shoulder and hip. This type of tape can be left on for several hours.

Kinesio Taping® (KT) was pioneered in Japan and uses specific specialized tapes and methods of taping; it too is reported to reduce pain while maintaining full range of motion. Kinesio Taping® can be left on for several days.

A technique not mentioned above is Functional Fascial Taping™ (FFT) pioneered by Ron Alexander. This is very similar to the McConnell style of taping but is used similarly to KT in that it is applied wherever pain is felt, and can be left on for days.

McConnell taping (MT), Kinesio Taping® (KT) and Functional Fascial Taping™ (FFT) have made progress in the area of pain management, especially with regards to application of the tape, but not necessarily how it works. MT, KT and FFT have common ground with regard to tape application; in comparison to the more traditional approach to taping (athletic taping),

relatively small amounts of tape are used and, in order for these types of techniques to be effective, it would seem that a certain amount of skin stretching needs to take place or a shortening between the two ends of the tape over the affected region (causing a corrugation effect on the skin). The direction in which the tape is applied may also play a role in how effective these types of tape jobs will be.

There is a growing body of evidence on all taping techniques, and research in this exciting area of therapy is ongoing. At present MT, KT and FFT, although widely used, still have a relatively smaller number of evidence-based research articles (with the possible exception of McConnell taping). However, the research that exists on all types of taping is very encouraging.

As stated in the introduction to this book, different techniques are used at different stages of repair and recovery. I will reiterate here that any area to be taped must be thoroughly examined and properly diagnosed. Any taping technique should be used as part of a comprehensive treatment and rehabilitation programme. It is up to the taper to decide which technique is used, when it is used and why it is used.

Tom Hewetson

REFERENCES

1. Casey KL. Neural mechanisms of pain. In: Carterette EC, Friedman MP (eds) Handbook of perception. New York: Academic Press, 1978: 183-219.

2. McConnell J. A novel approach to pain relief pre-therapeutic exercise. J Sci Med Sport 2000; 3: 325-334.

3. Hinman RS, Bennell KL, Crossley KM et al. Immediate effects of adhesive tape on pain and disability in individuals with knee osteoarthritis. Rheumatology 2003; 42: 865-869.

4. Vicenzino B, Brooksbank J, Minto J et al. Initial effects of elbow taping on pain-free grip strength and pressure pain threshold. J Orthop Sports Phys Ther 2003; 33: 400-407.

5. Kwon SS. The effects of the taping therapy on range of motion, pain and depression in stroke patient. Taehan Kanho Hakhoe Chi 2003; 33: 651-658.

6. Jeon MY, Jeong HC, Jeong MS et al. Effects of taping therapy on the deformed angle of the foot and pain in hallux valgus patients. Taehan Kanho Hakhoe Chi 2004; 34: 685-692.

7. Whittington M, Palmer S, MacMillan F. Effects of taping on pain and function in patellofemoral pain syndrome: a randomized controlled trial. J Orthop Sports Phys Ther 2004; 34: 504-510.

8. LaBella C. Patellofemoral pain syndrome: evaluation and treatment. Prim Care 2004; 31: 977-1003.

9. Lewis JS, Wright C, Green A. Subacromial impingement syndrome: the effect of changing posture on shoulder range of movement. J Orthop Sports Phys Ther 2005; 35: 72-87.

10. Aminaka N, Gribble PA. A systematic review of the effects of therapeutic taping on patellofemoral pain syndrome. J Athl Train 2005; 40: 341-351.

11. Hyland MR, Webber-Gaffney A, Choen L et al. Randomized controlled trial of calcaneal taping, sham taping, and plantar fascia stretching for the short-term management of plantar heel pain. J Orthop Sports Phys Ther 2006; 36: 364-371.

12. Radford JA, Landorf KB, Buchbinder R et al. Effectiveness of low-Dye taping for the short-term treatment of plantar heel pain: a randomised trial. BMC Musculoskelet Disord 2006; 9(7):64.

13. Callaghan MJ, Selfe J, McHenry A et al. Effects of patellar taping on knee joint proprioception in patients with patellofemoral pain syndrome. Man Ther 2008; 13(3): 192-199.

14. Hunter DJ, Zhang YQ, Niu JB et al. Patella malalignment, pain and patellofemoral progression: the Health ABC Study. Osteoarthritis Cartilage 2007; 15(10): 1120-1127.

15. Selfe J, Richards J, Thewlis D et al. The biomechanics of step descent under different treatment modalities used in patellofemoral pain. Gait Posture 2008; 27(2): 258-263.

16. Jaraczewska E, Long C. Kinesio taping in stroke: improving functional use of the upper extremity in hemiplegia. Top Stroke Rehabil 2006; 13: 31-42.

17. Panjabi MM. The stabilizing system of the spine: part 1, function, dysfunction, adaptation and enhancement. J Spinal Disord 1992; 5: 383-389.

18. Panjabi MM. The stabilizing system of the spine: part 2, neutral zone and instability hypothesis. J Spinal Disord 1992; 5: 390-396.

19. Dye SF. The knee as a biologic transmission with an envelope of function: a theory. Clin Orthop Relat Res 1996; 325: 10-18.

20. Dye SF, Vaupel GL, Dye CC. Conscious neurosensory mapping of the internal structures of the human knee without intraarticular anesthesia. Am J Sports Med 1998; 26: 773-777.

21. Dye SF. The pathophysiology of patellofemoral pain: a tissue homeostasis perspective. Clin Orthop Relat Res 2005; 436: 100-110.

Glossary

Anchor	Tape strips adhered directly to the skin to form a stable or secure base for subsequent tape strips.
Basketweave	An interlocking of three or more tape strands resembling a basket.
Bursa	A pouch or sack-like cavity made of synovium, containing synovial fluid, located at points of friction.
Butterfly	A series of overlapping taping strips with a typical form – wider at top and bottom, narrower in the middle.
Buttress	A prop or support used to strengthen a structure.
Capsule	A fibrous structure that envelops synovial joints.
Cartilage	A tough, elastic form of connective tissue found on articulating bony faces.
Caudal	Of or pertaining to the tail or posterior part of the body, as opposed to cranial.
Cranial	Of or pertaining to the skull or superior part of the body, as opposed to caudal.
Distal	Relatively remote from the centre of the body or point of attachment, as opposed to proximal.
Dorsal	Pertaining to the back or posterior/upper surface.
Figure of eight	A manoeuvre that consists of tracing the figure '8'.
Horizontal strip	A strip which is placed level with the horizon, as opposed to vertical strip.
Horseshoe	Padding made to resemble the 'U' shape of a horseshoe.
Inferior	Situated below or downward, as opposed to superior.
Lateral	Situated at or relatively near the outer side of the point of reference, as opposed to medial.
Ligament	A band of firm fibrous connective tissue forming a connection between bones, providing stability.
Lock	Any part that fastens, secures or holds something firmly in place.
Medial	Situated at or relatively near the middle of the point of reference, as opposed to lateral.
Plantar	Pertaining to the sole of the foot.
Proximal	Relatively near the central position of the body, as opposed to distal.
Stirrup	Any 'U'-shaped loop or piece.

Superior   Situated above or over another body part, as opposed to inferior.

Tendon   A cord of tough elastic connective tissue formed at the termination of a muscle, serving to transmit its force across a joint.

Vertical strip   A strip that is placed perpendicular to the line of the horizon, as opposed to horizontal strip.

Valgus   Deformities which displace the distal part of a joint away from the midline.

Varus   Deformities which displace the distal part of the joint towards the midline.

Volar   Pertaining to the palm of the hand.

Bibliography

1. American Medical Association, *Standard Nomenclature of Athletic Injuries* A.M.A., Chicago, USA, 1966.

2. Austin, Karin A., B.Sc.P.T., *Taping Booklet*. Physiothérapie International, Montreal, Canada, 1977.

3. Avis, Walter S., Editor, *Funk & Wagnalls Standard College Dictionary*. Fitzhenry & Whiteside Ltd., Toronto, Canada, 1978.

4. Backhouse, Kenneth M., O.B.E., V.R.D., and Hutchings R.T., *A Colour Atlas of Surface Anatomy*. Wolfe Medical Publications, London, UK, 1986.

5. Bouchard, Fernand, B.Sc. *Guide du soigneur*. Projet Perspective-Jeunesse, Montreal, Canada, 1972.

6. British Columbia Sports Medical Council, *British Columbia Sports Aid Program*, Victoria, B.C. Canada, 1984.

7. Cerney, J.V.M.D. *Complete Book of Athletic Taping Techniques*, Parker, New York, USA, 1972.

8. Cyriax, James, *Textbook of Orthopaedic Medical Diagnosis of Soft Tissue Injuries*. 8th Edition, Baillière Tindall, London, U.K, 1982

9. Dixon, Dwayne "Spike" A.T., *The Dixonary of Athletic Training*. Bloomcraft-Central Printing Inc., Bloomington, Indiana, USA, 1965.

10. Dominquez, Richard H., M.D., *The Complete Book of Sports Medicine*. Warner Books Inc., New York, USA. 1979.

11. Griffith, H. Winter, M.D., *Complete Guide to Sports Injuries*. The Body Press, HP Books Inc., Tucson, Arizona, USA, 1986.

12. Head, William F., M.S.F.,*Treatment of Athletic Injuries*. Frank W. Horner Ltd.; Montreal, Canada, 1966.

13. Hess, Heinrich, Prof.., *Sportverletzungen*. Luitpold-Werk, München (Munich), Germany, 1984.

14. Kapandji, I.A., *The Physiology of the Joints Vol 1 & 2*, Churchill Livingstone, Edinburgh, Scotland, 1970.

15. Logan, Gene A., Ph.D. R.P.T., and Logan, Roland F., *Techniques of Athletic Training*. Franklin-Adams Press, Pasadena, California, USA. 1959.

16. Magee, David J. *Orthopaedic Physical Assessment*, Saunders, Philadelphia, USA. 1987.

17. McConnell, J., B.App.Sc.(Phtg)., Grad.Dip., *The Management of Chrondromalacia Patellae: a long-term solution*, Physiotherapy, 32, (4), 1986, 215–223.

18. McMinn, R.M.H., and Hutchings, R.T., *A Colour Atlas of Human Anatomy*. Wolfe Publications, London, UK, 1977.

19. McMinn, R.M.H., Hutchings, R.T and Logan, B.M. *A Colour Atlas of Foot and Ankle Anatomy*. Wolfe Medical Publications, London, UK, 1982

20. Montag, Hans-Jürgen, and Asmussen, Peter D., *Functional Bandaging: A manual of bandaging technique*. Beiersdorf Bibliothek, Hamburg, Germany, 1981.

21. Reid, David C., *Sports Injury Assessment and Rehabilitation*, Churchill Livingstone, New York, USA, 1992.

22. Williams, Warwick (ed.) *Gray's Anatomy*. Churchill Livingstone, Edinburgh, Scotland, 1970.

23. Macdonald, Rose (ed) *Taping Techniques: Principles and Practice*. Butterworth Heinemann, London, UK, 2004.

24. Lederman, Eyal. *The Science and Practice of Manual Therapy*. Churchill Livingstone, London, UK, 2006.

T.E.S.T.S. chart listings

Index

INDEX